The
PRINCIPLED
PRACTICE

Cheryl A. Matschek, M.S.

Princess Publishing
Portland, Oregon

Published by:
Princess Publishing
P. O. Box 25406
Portland, OR 97225

Library of Congress Cataloging-in-Publication Data.

Matschek, Cheryl A.
    The principled practice: a comprehensive guide to the
    non-clinical aspects of dentistry/Cheryl A. Matschek.
        p. cm.
    ISBN 0-943367-05-0
    1. Dentistry--Practice.   2. Dental offices--Management.
    3. Dental offices--Personnel Management.   I. Title.
    RK58.M346   1995
    617'.0068--dc20   94-47411
                                                            CIP

Printed in the United States of America
First Printing 1995

To my loving husband, Norm,
who fills my life with joy
as we make the journey together.
You are a blessing to your patients,
and to all those who know you.
Thank you for your support of and belief
in me, and for loving me through
this process.
You are always an inspiration to me
and I love you.

To my mother, Cecile Hammill.
By your example you have
given me the love of people and of medicine.
You are an incredible example of commitment,
persistence, determination, enthusiasm,
spirit, integrity and leadership.
You have given so much to medicine
and all the lives you have touched along
the way, and most certainly mine.
I have always loved you.

To our team: Judy, Linda and Tami.
You are incredible.
You are the team that
everyone hopes and prays for...
and I love each of you.
Thank you for being such
an important part of my life.

CONTENTS

Contents

Part Three
You and Your Patients: Building Your Practice

Foreword

I feel privileged to write the foreword for this book, and especially honored, for I am married to the author.

Every once in a while someone comes along who makes a tremendous difference in our lives. I am happy to say that Cheryl has made a magnificent difference in my life, both personally and professionally. I met Cheryl when she was introduced by a mutual friend who knew I was looking for a consultant to do an analysis for my dental practice. That was the beginning, and what was to follow changed the course of my life in so many wonderful, positive ways.

I've never known anyone who has such an incredible knowledge of so many facets of life and business today, or who has such a great understanding of the systems and the people aspects of dentistry (or any other business for that matter) as Cheryl. Nor do I know of anyone else who has such a tremendous desire and ability to help other people and organizations grow and develop.

Cheryl has been consistently sought after for keynotes and training throughout the world since she began speaking professionally in 1979. As you read this book I think you'll understand why. She is dynamic, enthusiastic, high energy...and has a beautiful spirit.

You are in for an adventure! Within this book is a wealth of information and how-to's for making your practice come alive. You'll learn about yourself and your leadership responsibilities, as well as how to carry them out. You'll have all you need to establish the direction you want to head. You'll learn how to build, train, motivate, and compensate that "dream team" most of us have dreamed about, but have never experienced. You'll learn about sales and marketing, again something most of us have never really mastered. She'll help you understand the practice from the patient's point of view, and help you to position yourself for greater patient relations. In short, you will get all the benefits of a master of human relations and human potential in a book you will refer to time and time again.

I've watched the entire process of this valuable book being "born." Cheryl has worked around the clock at times, written while

I was out on the golf course or gone fishing, while we were travelling on business or for vacation, and in the hotel room of whatever town she was speaking in, to make this available for you. Because of her dedication and commitment to her work and those she serves, she has lovingly and caringly poured out her wisdom and guidance. If you will listen carefully to what she has to say, you will be touched and transformed as I was and continue to be.

As you read this, you'll most likely feel Cheryl is talking directly to you...and she is. Create in yourself an open channel as you read, and a deep inner knowing will rise from your relationship to it. Listen to it. Let it come forth from within. And then, act from your integrity on what results.

I know you will learn from The Principled Practice and enjoy it. But what I hope you will do is use what you learn. The truths, the principles that Cheryl will give you can set you free and make your practice a most productive and satisfying place to work...for you, and for your practice team.

I proudly present to you my wife, Cheryl Matschek.

J. Norman Matschek, D.M.D.
Portland, Oregon

Preface

There is no perfect practice, and every practice has room for improvement. That's why this book was written. We are entering an exciting, dramatic time in dentistry where much is changing rapidly and there is no indication that it will slow down, and certainly it will not stop.

Technology is running ahead faster than we can keep pace. Information systems are moving toward us with ever increasing speed. On-line, real-time systems for developing links between practices, insurance companies, universities, clinical centers, think tanks, data bases...and who knows what else...has not only knocked on our doors, but already made entry. What we experience in dentistry in the years ahead will be much different than today, especially as it relates to diagnostics and treatment.

To be effective in this rapidly changing, dynamic world of dentistry, will require the ability to lead and to develop people. More than any other area of your practice, leadership is needed if you are to handle and cope effectively with the multitude of changes and opportunities that will be yours. And that is why this book is written. When we are clear about our vision, mission and values, when we have a dedicated, committed, well-trained team working together synergistically, and when we understand the principles of selling...then we will have what is necessary to build the practice of our dreams...regardless of the outside circumstances.

At this point in our development, when change is coming so fast, it is not a question of do we like it, but how will we deal with it. Few are comfortable with change, but *not changing is not an option*. Where we will be in dentistry five or ten or fifteen years from today will certainly not be where we are today. That's a given. Are we strong enough to deal with this change...this transformation? Yes and No. It depends upon the practice; it depends upon the leader; and it depends upon the team the leader has developed.

Will Rogers once said, "Even if you're on the right track, you'll get run over if you just sit there." To feel comfortable no longer means finding a safe place to conduct our business and maintain the status quo. No, the only way to feel comfortable today is to become comfortable with, and make a friend of change. It is here to stay. Responding to change can be mystifying, exasperating, exciting, depressing, fearful, dynamic, or all of the above at once! Many people tend to resist the changes that give the greatest results or make the greatest contribution to the practice, because they are often personal changes. That's because it requires going outside our comfort zone. And yet, change is what allows us to experience growth and advancement and success.

How to you respond to change? How does your staff respond to change? Either you will accept it and move forward with it, knowing it is your path to the future, or you will resist it and fight it at every turn. And your staff, in most circumstances, will accept or reject, work with, or resist change based on your response to the changes affecting dentistry and your practice in particular. Certainly your response will be up to you. You have the power of choice to greet it with positive expectation, or you can choose to bemoan the change and find yourself fighting it at every turn. The ability to respond with positive expectation demands that the element of leadership becomes an everyday part of the practice.

Many dentists are in practices today that they would like to grow. And some are growing, but many more are growing very slowly, if at all. In fact, many practices are actually declining when you take into account the value of the dollar and inflation. So what do you do? How do you stay in front. How can you maximize your possibilities?

The answer is not simple, nor will it happen overnight. It has to do with new paradigms, new belief systems. It means coming to view your practice from a different perspective and acquiring some skills that perhaps are a bit foreign to you. These are skills not taught in most dental schools today, and certainly were not in the past. We can all answer the question of how good we are. None of us, however, can answer how good we can be. There is so much more ahead on our journey.

Before we move into Part One, stop for a moment and make a list of the pro's and con's of your practice. What do you really like about your practice? What would you like to change? Where do you feel something is missing? Invest the time right now to ask yourself these questions, and then refer to these regularly throughout the book.

We are blessed. We choose our path and thereby create our reality. If you don't like what you are receiving, what is coming into your life and your practice right now, maybe it is time to look at your life, at your programming, and at your potential...then make some changes and move forward.

One of the practice shifts is that dental insurance, as we have known it, will most likely end. Within the next several years the benefits offered to employees by employers will be squeezed to the point that only medical and pension type contributions will be made. In fact, to go around the benefits paid to employees, many employers are moving toward the direction of associating themselves with part-time help and independent contractors. As dental insurance takes a backseat it will be a great opportunity for you to learn to attract those patients who truly want the services you offer. It means your team must be more committed than ever before, and have greater skills than ever before.

The latest statistics indicate that 50 percent of Americans do not have a regular dentist. This should be exciting to us and give us hope and encouragement about the potential for our practices!

The Principled Practice was written with all this in mind. It was written with all the team members in mind, but specifically directed to the doctor. Unless changes begin here the rest can't happen. One thing I know for certain: by working with the principles and processes communicated in this book, by living them every day, you will transform your practice into one that is more successful, where the team is happy and productive, and you will all feel satisfied, fulfilled and enthusiastic about dentistry.

Now, I hope my efforts and energy will truly make a positive difference in your life, as well as your practice. Join me on the journey, we've only just begun.

Part One

You and Your Practice: The Doctor as Leader

Chapter 1

PRINCIPLES

Universal principles control our lives. These are the principles of success, as well as the principles of mediocrity...depending upon our response to them. They have been with us since the beginning. They have never changed! When we are in tune with these principles operating in our lives, we will produce incredible results and a great deal of personal peace and satisfaction.

Universal principles are the laws of cause and effect that operate every day, for every person, in every time and every situation. They are not situational, applied to one particular circumstance but not in another. They show us that what we sow, we also shall reap. These laws of the universe are balanced, and we cannot disturb that balance without feeling the negative effects in our own lives. When we pay attention to these principles our dental practices will thrive, as well as our personal well-being, financial well-being and personal relationships.

As we begin this journey through *The Principled Practice* it is important not to compare yourself to the doctor or practice next door. One size does not fit all! No two people are exactly alike...and no two practices are exactly alike. What is important is that you sincerely question and delve into your values, vision, and mission to make sure you are headed in the right direction for you. It takes discernment and listening to determine what is really the most appropriate for your practice. You can chart your own course, travel your own path, and as a result choose your own destiny. The answers you are looking for will only come by having the courage to question, and then to choose, what feels "at home" for your practice.

When a patient presents a painful situation, in order to make a meaningful diagnosis and recommendation for treatment, you must get at the cause of the pain. The same goes for our personal and professional lives. In order to make a real difference, we need to get at the cause of the problem, concern, or dissatisfaction. Understanding the principles operating in our lives will help us to do just that.

There is no magic formula for success. If there was we would all adopt it right now and head for the bank. But we are not all the same. We don't practice the same. Our values may not be the same. *But the principles never change.* Certainly there are many, many principles operating in our lives every moment. The following, however, are those identified as being extraordinarily important to realizing the results of *The Principled Practice.*

• **Belief Systems.** We cannot experience something that is outside the boundaries of our current belief. We must open ourselves and empty ourselves of old beliefs and assumptions before there is room for something new.

• **Energy.** Energy flows to where our concentration goes. We attract what we are, not what we like! Whatever we put out is what we will get back. The law of cause and effect is involved here. Every cause must have a certain, definite effect. We reap what we sow with exact precision. We live in a world of interconnectedness...nothing is isolated. Every event is linked to the onebefore.

• **Intention.** Matter follows mind...as you think, so you become. Thoughts are things. You get what you get because of the thoughts you think and the energy you send forth and draw back as a result. Whatever we send out in thought or intention will return to us. What we resists, persists. What we hold in thought comes true in our experience. *We manifest on the outside what is going on in the inside.* We create the visible conditions outside us that most resonate with our inner state of being.

• **Integrity.** Integrity is the balance between values and moments of truth. How will I act in this moment? Integrity means living out what you say you believe and hold as important. It is walking your talk.

• **Synergy.** You will accomplish more as a team than when you act independently.

• **Responsibility.** Every person is ultimately responsible for his or her own life. You, doctor, are also responsible for your own practice and its success (or lack of).

• **Trust.** This is an integral part of character and involves keeping commitments.

• **Order.** Order is the first law of expansion.

• **Balance.** Without balance in our life, we will ultimately be met with dissatisfaction, stress, and a lack of fulfillment.

• **Ethics.** You cannot have harmony without a commitment to ethical behavior.

• **Discipline.** Discipline provides a constancy from day to day, independent from how the day is going or what happened the day before.

• **Attraction.** There is no scarcity in the universe, only abundance. Abundance is not something we manufacture, but something we open ourselves to and accept. We receive that which we are willing to let in, but we block ourselves with belief in scarcity. You can have anything you want when you develop the consciousness to receive it. Whatever you focus your thought on expands. Abundance will never be a factor of how much money you have. Rather, it is always a factor of how you *feel* about what money you have.

• **Service.** Only what you give, ultimately, will be returned.

When we live by these thirteen principles, we will *respond* based on those principles rather than *react* based on circumstances, situation or emotions. When we live by principles we take control of our life. We are no longer victims. We are not controlled by our past or what was. Instead, we are moving in the direction of our ability to choose. It is true that we cannot always control the situation, but we can control our choices....and when that choice, in the best of times or the worst, is based on principles, we can be sure it is for our highest and best good, and for the highest and best good for all those involved.

Because these principles are not situational, we find we can only be effective to the degree that we understand and work in harmony with them moment by moment. They operate in the universe without regard to any person...and in regard to every person. When we listen to our inner voice, and respond in harmony with these principles, we are acting with integrity. When we work with them, not against them, we will see our lives change dramatically for the better. We will literally open the floodgates to receive all that is good.

Obedience precedes authority. The law obeys us when we obey the natural laws or principles, just as the law of electricity must be obeyed before the power of electricity is at our disposal. If it is misunderstood or misapplied, disaster is inevitable. So it is with universal principles.

What we're talking about in *The Principled Practice* is a journey...not a destination. Every principle is something we live each and every day. Every time you unlock the door to your practice and open for business...every time a practice team member picks up the telephone...every time you interact with a patient or an employee...every time you greet a patient.....the principles are working, either for you or against you, depending upon your thoughts and behavior.

These principles must be the basis of goals, decisions and strategies. As a result, a *single standard of conduct* needs to be employed throughout our lives...both publicly and privately. The abundance you desire (both materially and spiritually) will come as a result of definite principles. If you lack in some area it is not because of what you do....but in truth because of what *causes* you to do what you do...your motives, your intentions, your beliefs, your values...in short, the principles you live by.

> When we abandon the principles,
> we are the ones that suffer, not the principle.

We cannot have a healthy, functioning team when we put up with garbage. We cannot live in the present moment when we are living in the past or in the future. We can't ask for what we want when we will accept and live with what we don't want. We cannot love when we live in fear. We cannot learn to be trusting when we are constantly in the process of defending and protecting ourselves. And, we cannot see what is right when we are continually focusing on what is wrong. We must make choices...for certain things cannot exist simultaneously. And, we will make choices based on our values, whether or not we are aware of the principles that will influence the results of those choices.

Ultimately, knowledge of and understanding of these principles give us hope for the future and power for the present, and *principled action* will keep us in harmony with the principles and on a purposeful path even when the path may seem unclear.

The principled practice is always clear about its focus and direction. Without guiding principles, we will have a "situational practice"; there will be a lack of cohesiveness, integration, interdependence, and consistency. Teamwork is virtually impossible, synergism is not inherent because people are not capable of a sustained response when they don't know the focus. Without principles, leadership is almost sure to be non-existent or haphazard at best. Without principles, a practice with a stated mission most likely will have difficulty in carrying out that mission.

Have you noticed that no matter where you go or how fast you are running there is really no running away from anything? That you carry what it is you are running from with you? That sooner or later the things you don't want to deal with catch up with you? The underlying thinking is that the problems we have, the challenges in our life...personally and professionally...lie outside us in the circumstances, the other people, the location, etc. Too often our lives aren't working because we quit working at life. We forget that *we* must take responsibility. There is no other way, at least not for very long.

Remember, as we invest this time together, that life is a journey, not a destination...and it's how we make the journey that counts. Welcome to the journey! Sit back, make yourself comfortable and explore with me the principles and actions that will allow you to develop the practice of your dreams. First stop, leadership.

Chapter 2

LEADERSHIP

Dentistry has changed from what we have known in the past. Equipment and materials are different. What our patients want and expect is different. Our employees are different. Therefore, in order to stand out and give our employees and our patients a reason to stay with us, what we do, we must do *differently and better.* In the past we could practice successfully with good management. Today, management is not enough. It takes quality leadership. Leadership can make or break the practice. It can be the factor that determines whether the practice will be mediocre, marginally successful, or highly successful.

One question I am continually asked is, "What sort of leadership style is more effective?" And I have only one answer: supportive. Supportive leadership is the only kind of leadership there is...otherwise it is not leadership. Supportive leadership is leadership from the heart...with a heart. Leadership is helping people discover their unique personal characteristics. It's creating an atmosphere where people rekindle desire and become willing to utilize their strengths. Leadership is purposeful influence that takes a team some place good, but where they have never before been. It is about creating workplaces that trust and honor and encourage the full expression of ourselves. Leadership is understanding that without effective, motivated people, tasks and job descriptions won't be completed as effectively as they could be. It is about supporting one another in all our experiences: risks and rewards, uncertainties and confidences, sadness and joys, triumphs and defeats.

This period of transformation we are in will carry us well into the next millennium. As part of that transformation we are beginning to understand the wealth of potential that remains untapped in the most important asset we have in our practices....our people. Leadership requires that we be willing and desirous of building our team members. It requires that we be willing to step out of the comfort zone to risk and change in order to grow. We do not have the luxury of staying with what we've always done, even though it may have worked well in the past. If we try to maintain what has always been, we will inevitably begin the process of decline. The questions still remain, however: Where are we headed? How will we get there? How do we unlock the potential?

These are the cornerstones upon which leadership is built today. The Stanford Research Institute, Harvard, and the Carnegie Foundation have conducted independent studies indicating that 85% of success in business depends on people skills. Technical skills and other abilities make up only 15% of the determining factors of success. Simply stated, when you know how to make your patients and your staff feel good about you, and the experience of working with and doing business with you, your success potential has increased tremendously.

Consciously or subconsciously, people today are seeking ways to be fulfilled, to find wholeness of self, to be connected to something of importance... something that makes a difference. The leader has the power to help make this search productive and rewarding by the environment that is created in the practice. When this is accomplished the result is happier, more fulfilled individuals who produce more, care more, and will lead the practice to even greater productivity and profitability. We are all seeking purpose and meaning in our lives. Leadership is about encouraging others to become their very best, to tap into their potential, to discover that greater meaning and feeling of making a difference.

Leadership of days gone by was based, to a great extent, on fear and intimidation. But that's not real leadership. The *Principled Practice* requires leadership that is encouraging and inspires team members to excellence without intimidation and fear. It expresses an ethic of self-development for all members of the practice to become the best they can be. Leaders understand the theory of the self-fulfilling prophecy and realize that people have a way of becoming what they are encouraged to become...not what we tell them to become or force them to become.

Leadership for the 21st century means connecting hearts with heads. It means being vulnerable...activating your emotions so you can activate your team members...and then your patients. It means speaking your experience from the heart so you touch your team and patients with your passion....and then they will follow. Leadership is about leading ourselves and those with whom we work to a different place...a place centered in knowing that we are much more than what we see on the outside...and in believing in the potential we each possess. It is about creating workplaces of trust and empowerment so the fullness of who we are can be expressed.

Three principles are important here:

Leadership is learned. No one is a born leader. Leadership cannot be taught, but the principles can be taught. Once understood, they must be put into practice to actually learn them and know them.

Leadership is a journey, a process. You never become a leader once and for all. Leadership is always an active process of becoming.

The true leader understands that success is a result of enriching the lives of others...it does not come at the expense of them. The true leader understands that people with whom they work want respect and acceptance. The leader gives that respect and helps others awaken to and tap into their "as yet" untapped potential. The leader knows that to profit by walking over people, trampling them in the process and using them, is not to succeed at all.

Four Pre-requisites to Leadership

Before we can discuss the characteristics of the leader, there are four pre-requisites we must understand and be willing to accept. These pre-requisites are necessary for any leader. A leader must:

1.   Have a clear sense of purpose. This requires understanding values, vision, mission and goals. These will be discussed in the following chapters.

Reviewing leadership and management of the past reveals that many have managed themselves, their homes and their businesses reactively, after the fact, correcting mistakes. Leadership, however, requires proactive behavior. This is much like the prevention you practice in dentistry.

2.   Know thyself. A leader must know how to develop leaders, motivate people, and counsel them. This requires knowing yourself first, and is an essential ingredient in gaining the support of the team. Understanding how your own mind works is important. The paradigms, or patterns of thinking, can be bridges or barriers to communication and relationships. Just as Socrates said, "know thyself," the true leader also understands the importance of "knowing thyself."

One of the hardest things for us to do is look objectively and realistically at ourselves without deception, without losing hope, and without self-glorification. When we look at ourselves honestly we will become much more effective as leaders and managers, we will have a greater influence on others, and we will have better interpersonal relationships. As a result we will find greater personal satisfaction and fulfillment.

Understanding yourself will also help you understand the behavioral tendencies of other people so you can communicate with them in such a way that they will understand what you are trying to say. This is extremely important once you understand that other people are not necessarily motivated by the same things you are. By understanding your team's behavioral and personality characteristics you will be better able to build on their strengths.

3. Plan. Once you know where you are headed, you must determine how you are going to get there. Leaders have the vision, they dream, and then they determine what it will take to turn that vision into reality. They develop the strategy, with the help of their team. They have goals and objectives that are both attainable and realistic.

4. Implement. Once the plan is identified, leaders move forward with the implementation. The leader understands that the moment of absolute certainty may never arrive.

Each of these four pre-requisites is a necessary and vital function of a leader. Let's look at the characteristics of a leader.

Characteristics of Leaders

Although this entire book deals with leadership, there are many characteristics that identify a true leader. Every person has at least the spark of the these qualities somewhere within. The development of these characteristics takes desire, commitment and practice, but they are worth the effort. Not only are these important to your practice, but they will serve you well in every area of your life.

Visionary. Leaders develop vision, values, purpose and mission...and will challenge tradition if it is necessary to proactively work towards the future. They don't sit back, waiting for life to happen. Rather, leaders take responsibility for their own lives. They are solution-oriented, not problem-oriented. They have a vision. Without vision, there is no leadership.

Flexible and able to handle change. The only constant is change. We don't have to like it, but we must understand it. It is deadly to be apathetic toward the changes coming in our industry and close our eyes to them. Leaders realize that what worked well for the practice in the past may not be the products, services, and ways of doing business that will be the most productive today and in the future. To be successful today requires the ability to adapt to changing situations and to anticipate as much as possible the opportunities, as well as the challenges, just over the horizon. This requires that a leader be flexible enough to change. To be strong, we must be flexible. Just as any building without "give" cannot withstand an earthquake of any size, neither can an individual withstand the test of leadership without being flexible.

Marilyn Ferguson, in *The Aquarian Conspiracy*, said, "No one can persuade another to change. Each of us guards a gate of change that can only be opened from the inside. We cannot open the gate of another, either by argument or emotional appeal." Being flexible means being open to new ideas.

People change in one of two ways...impact or repetition. Impact can be devastating because we have no time to prepare, but it does have its upside. Since we have no time to adjust or procrastinate, many of our options are removed and we are forced to deal with the change immediately. Planned change, however, gives us the opportunity to think through the alternatives and decide what we believe is best at any given time for a particular situation.

We must become masters of change, masters of renewal. This means learning to be comfortable with being uncomfortable because there is most always a period during a transition when it is not comfortable. And we can only do that in a supportive environment...one that supports the team as well as the doctor.

Identify the needs of their people, then treat them equally, but differently. Leaders are enthusiastic about creating an atmosphere that will bring out the best in others. They understand that the only way to relate to team members individually requires knowing their people. They spend time with their teams and study the individuals within the team. They work to identify what motivates each individual and what the fears are. They work from the inside and look to where a person is headed. They want to know what makes them tick so they can support them, encourage their strengths, and help them develop personal power. They ask questions like:

How would you like to change?
What would it take for you to feel fulfilled and really happy?
Where have you been?
Where are you going?
What do you believe?

Where are your sore spots, hurts, places that need healing?
What do you like (love).....dislike (fear)?
What do you value?
What about dentistry do you really like? Dislike?

The winning situation occurs when the leader finds out what the individuals want and then incorporates that into the practice plan so the employees can reach their individual goals while at the same time meeting the practice goals.

We have, for too long, treated many employees as a resource that was plentiful, cheap and always expendable. Instead of looking to people as our most important resource, the attention was given to increasing productivity and profitability through new technology and better systems. Today's employees, even if it doesn't appear so on the surface, want the opportunity to work in a position and practice where they can *invest* themselves to use their full human potential. They want to make a difference. They want to be valued for the individuals they are and the difference they can make.

Consider each of your employees. Does this desire seem to be missing? If so, keep looking. Most likely it has been covered over by many layers of protective coating because of past experiences and the fear of being vulnerable, embarrassed, or hurt. If this is the situation, the individual may not even recognize or know where her desire is herself. When you are willing and care enough to help each of your employees find that spark of aliveness and desire, not only will they benefit and blossom into the wonderful people they can be, but you will reap the benefits in many, many ways.

Risk takers. They create an atmosphere where failures or mistakes are not fatal or final. *The ability to take risks is the willingness to fail in order to succeed.* In order to become good at anything, one must first be willing to do whatever it is many times poorly until the skill is developed to do it well. That's the way we learn anything. Probably the first time you took an impression in dental school you didn't do it as well as you do today. Isn't that right? As we grow, change, and are confronted with new ways of doing things, we are back in dental school, so to speak. We must begin somewhere, and sometimes that means making mistakes to get where we are going.

Plan your risks. If you feel it is helpful, do the two column approach Ben Franklin often used. What are the pros and cons of this risk? If the pros outweigh the cons, move forward. Make a plan B for the cons. What will I do if this happens? You can reduce your fear to near zero with a plan to deal with the possible cons.

The only practices that are successful today and will maintain the edge of success for tomorrow will be the ones that allow at least a few mistakes in the growing process. It is impossible to innovate, grow, expand and progress without making some mistakes. Sometimes, however, we don't give ourselves the room to admit mistakes and instead we attempt to prove our "okayness" through our "false perfection." This inability to admit mistakes does three things: it continues our self-deception, interrupts our relationships with others, and teaches others that it is not okay to make mistakes. This only leads downhill to increased problems, decreased productivity and fulfillment, and stagnation.

When we create an environment where people are afraid of making mistakes (because of the reprimands that follow) or admitting mistakes, we have also created an environment that stifles, and eventually snuffs out, the spark within each individual that turns potential into reality. We have inspired fear, not confidence. When this happens the most likely result will be an employee who is afraid to act for fear of making another mistake and receiving another reprimand.

Accepting risks and mistakes as a part of the learning process means creating a *fear-free learning environment* where the only stupid questions are the ones not asked and where everyone is regarded as equal, but different. We need these fear-free environments to give our people the opportunity to practice without fear of reprisal when an honest mistake is made. Remember: We learn from mistakes. Getting it right is often simply the result of practice, of doing something enough times until we get it right.

When your people have dealt with rejection or failure, or have stepped out and risked and subsequently made a mistake, be there to help them pick up the pieces and maintain their self-esteem. Help them to learn from the mistakes so they can benefit from them and grow in the process. Your employees need to know you are on their side working *with them*, not against them. They need to know you delight in finding them doing what it takes to grow...and that means occasional mistakes. Cheer them on, persuade them to take one more step. Put them back in the pool before fear takes over and they recoil from ever swimming again.

Establish high standards and expectations that are realistic *and achievable.* People are not inspired when nothing is expected of them. They are not inspired by *just good enough* or *mediocrity.* This means that leaders expect the best from their people. If you don't, it won't be long before the team is impacted negatively, the motivation declines, creativity and desire to go the extra mile is weakened, and you lose commitment to the practice. The power of expectations is great.

Throw out the bell curve mentality and draw forth a new paradigm. We have for too long clung to the concept that a certain percentage of people will make it no matter what, another percentage will never make it regardless, and those in the middle will make it if they have the right tools and environment. All of this is learned and has to do with our mental models...our ways of thinking. It is amazing what a person can and will do if they know you believe in them and believe they can. Don't limit your employees by your own limited thinking.

Integrity and character. It takes a whole life to build character and one minute to lose it. I've heard it said that the real measure of character is what you would do if you knew you'd never get caught. Character is what you control about yourself.

What do you say you stand for? What do you say you value? What do you say you do for your employees? And do you do it? When we act with integrity we come from the totality of who we are and are remarkably effective. Integrity means walking the talk...and when we do, we provide the model for our employees to do the same.

Leaders must have a strong belief system to deal with today's challenges and maintain the courage of their convictions. They must be morally strong. The principles of truth, honesty, and justice...without being judgmental...are essential.

James Allen, well known author of *As A Man Thinketh* wrote, "From the state of a man's heart proceed the conditions of his life;

his thoughts blossom into deeds, and his deeds bear the fruitage of character and destiny."

Decision makers. Deciding is often more difficult than carrying through after you have made the decision, but leaders recognize that not making a decision is in itself a decision to let things happen by default, or let circumstances dictate the choice. Indecision wastes time, money, energy, talent and often involves missed opportunities. The ability to have confidence in your decisions is equally important.

Leaders know they don't have to make decisions in a vacuum. In fact, when they enlist the team in the process the decisions will be supported much more readily. Certainly not every decision in the practice should involve the team, but when it is appropriate you will find they'll not only come up with ideas that are tremendous and you might never have thought of yourself, but they will feel much more an integral part of the practice. This brings with it a greater feeling of fulfillment and satisfaction, resulting in increased productivity.

Have a sense of humor. This doesn't mean taking things lightly, but it does mean keeping things in perspective. There is an old saying, "If you take yourself too seriously, no one else will!" Leaders have fun and can turn routine tasks into pleasurable or enjoyable experiences. This includes being able to express feelings and lighten the load of all with whom they associate.

Have fun together in your team. People love to have fun, but many have forgotten how. Especially in the workplace! We have mistaken being "professional" for being stodgy, serious, no-nonsense, solemn , stuffy, and even uppity. This is far from the meaning of professional. When fun is a part of the workplace you will find team members going the extra mile over and over again.

Positive and expectant. Much of the team members motivation is stimulated by the leader and leaders understand this. Leaders are hope-filled and keep their own motivation high. They realize that 90% of what they do is attitude, leading to success, failure or mediocrity. Enthusiastic doctors create enthusiastic staff, and enthusiastic patients as a result. Leaders have the ability to see the sun behind the cloud, the light beyond the shadow, the expanse beyond the horizon. They can see the opportunity in the obstacles, the good in a difficult situation, the hope when others don't, and they can maintain their faith when others have lost theirs. Sometimes, the leader is the one carrying the candle when all the other candles have gone out...lighting the way until the flame can be rekindled within the individual.

Aware of what power is and use it wisely. True power is the ability to create an environment that motivates, loves, encourages, and helps people recognize their uniqueness and potential. Leaders don't judge people by the "obvious cover," but understand that sometimes what seems obvious is simply an extraordinary cloak for something absolutely incredible.

Several years ago I was in the market for a new car, but hadn't decided what I wanted to purchase. One Saturday morning I stopped by a dealership I hadn't yet visited to see if anything really grabbed my attention. As I drove into the lot, I noticed a car I hadn't seen before. (It was the first year for the Toyota Supra.) Not even knowing what it was, I knew I wanted that car.

I got out of my car, walked up to the Supra parked directly in front of the showroom, and peered in the window. Watching from the showroom window were seven salesmen standing around drinking coffee. Not one of them made any effort to come in my direction.

Dressed in jeans and sweatshirt, and appearing much younger than my age, I walked in the showroom. Another salesman, walking toward the showroom from the lounge, was the only person who approached me! After I asked for a test drive he promptly grabbed the keys and away we went. Not one of the other seven put one foot forward in my direction!

I can't help but feel that the only reason I wasn't approached by the other salesmen (how often does one walk onto an automobile lot and remain unapproached by a salesperson?) is that they thought I didn't "look like a qualified prospect." I looked too young, and wasn't dressed in clothes that suggested I had the funds necessary for the purchase. What a mistake on their part! The last gentlemen, who did pay attention to me, made a nice sale and I was on my way off the lot with a new Supra! The moral, obviously, is not to judge a book by its cover.

Leaders understand this principle and keep themselves open to others without judging. In your dental practice this means with both the employees and the patients. How many times have we pre-judged what a patient could afford, and adjusted the recommended treatment plan accordingly? (We'll discuss this further in Part III.)

Using power wisely means taking responsibility for using it in ways that uplift and encourage others. It means believing that each individual is worthwhile, and treating them as though they really matter. This includes every human being with whom we come into contact...not just employees, patients, or authority figures.

Committed. Leaders follow through in spite of obstacles. They take one day at a time, continually moving forward in the direction of their goals. Being committed means transforming the promise into reality. We can speak loudly and often of what our intentions might be, but it is our commitment that leads to follow through...and this speaks much louder than any words.

Good communicators. Communication is the key to every successful relationship...with patients, employees and every other person with whom we come into contact. There can be no leadership without developing the skills of good communication.

Team builders. Leaders place great importance on teamwork. The dental practice operates in such a way that individuals must work together in order to function effectively. When you create an atmosphere that builds a cohesive unit, a team, you will have not only doubled your capacity to produce, but the synergism created increases it exponentially.

The team also creates the environment that provides a sense of belonging. For some people, work is their main (and for some the only) source of identity and companionship. Many people will stay with a practice where they find this sense of team, of belonging, of making a difference, even if they could go somewhere else and be paid a higher salary or hourly wage.

Trust their people. Trusting doesn't mean that you never inspect what is being accomplished. In fact a very important principle is to *inspect what you expect.* This is all part of being accountable.

If you really feel you can't trust your employees, each and every one of them, then perhaps the person you cannot trust should not be a part of your practice. Certainly without trust, and in the environment of suspicion, encouragement *cannot* and *will not* happen. Neither will commitment or loyalty of your team members. When you love your people, believe in them and stand up for them. When you do you will find a team who will be loyal to the end.

Leaders are also trustworthy. They tell people the truth. They admit not having all the answers and ask for help in reaching workable solutions.

Provide strong, visible support of their people. This will not and cannot happen without trust. Leaders support their people rather than force them. They will work through their people, not over them. They understand that patience and nurturing of employees will gain support for the entire team, as well as the practice. In fact, the more supportive the leader, the more the employees will identify with and support the vision, mission and goals to be achieved.

Service. Part of trusting your people is backing them by service and full visible support. Someone once said that every person seeking to balance the law of life should first seek to render service. Leaders are not afraid to serve. They help their people grow in whatever ways they can. They reach down and pull their people up beside them, not jealous or afraid that the employee may rise to greater heights and leave. Instead, leaders help their people to become all they are capable of becoming.

Life-long learners. The old model of leadership has shifted. It was once based on the belief that the average person lacks power and personal vision, and was incapable of dealing with change. Today's view of leadership is quite different. Leaders are responsible for building practices where people are inspired and motivated to learn for a lifetime, to grow day by day, to become all they were created to become. That requires life-long learning.

Re-evaluate yourself often. Just as you do reviews with your people, find out how you are doing. *Leadership is not an ego game. One way to evaluate yourself is to ask your team members how you are doing. What three things do I do in leading/managing our team that you like and feel I should do more of? What three things do I do that you don't like and feel I should do less of?* It takes a big person to do this, but a leader is a big person.

Scary? Perhaps. But only because we're not used to opening ourselves up for feedback at the top.

Model the behavior and attitudes they want and expect. It is difficult, if not impossible, to teach principles without modeling. It isn't good enough to simply talk the talk, telling them what you expect, and not expecting that from yourself as well.

What your team sees you doing day in and day out will send a more convincing message about what is important to you than anything you could ever tell them, or any motto you might employ. The way you treat your patients, suppliers, peers, and employees is what sets the "real" rules in the practice. In other words, *you are the message.* This goes for how you respect time commitments, follow through on what you say you will do, as well as the many personal characteristics including honesty and sincerity.

Leadership requires loyalty. In order to have loyalty from your team, you must first be loyal to them. Loyalty doesn't come with the title of owner or leader, it must be earned. Without loyalty from the leader there will be little commitment from the team, and commitment is critical in order to create the synergism necessary for maximum results. Commitment cannot be dictated, commanded, or regulated...it must be inspired. It takes a leader to create an environment where this commitment is forthcoming. Unless you are loyal to your team members, you will not gain the commitment necessary from your team to make the journey towards your vision.

Principled Leadership is love made manifest. Leaders are *love made manifest* in their being, in their existence. Leaders recognize that in order to love others, they must first love themselves. They must be comfortable with themselves and have no need to try to be someone else. They realize that the more real they are, the more authentic they become, the more genuine is their expression and communication, the more people will be able to relate to them. It is in this environment that team members feel much safer to express themselves. Loving allows this.

These twenty characteristics will determine how effective you will be as a leader. They will insure that you are a supportive, encouraging leader. Leadership that encourages and builds people leads with the heart...and guides with the head. The heart is about values and the *principled leader* has clearly identified what values are important...and lives them out daily. Leading with the heart means making the heart connection. When you lead from the heart you will touch your staff and patients with your passion....and when you do, they will follow.

Leadership is a Way of Life

Leadership is a way of life. This means that leadership is not a situational ethic. Instead, leaders are leaders all the time, whether at the office or on the golf course, at home or in a social setting. This doesn't mean they are not followers...in fact leaders in one situation may be followers in another situation. That does not, however, change the fact that they are leaders, and all the characteristics we have discussed still apply.

Leadership is About "Being"

For so long we have been rebuilding, restructuring, rearranging, and redoing. It is time to stop...and to *begin by being*. That's from the heart. *When you change the letters around in begin....you get being.* That's what leadership is about. It is about *being* first, and *doing* second, as a result of that being. The practice will draw from your spiritual energy all that it needs to move toward your vision.

So many people go through life with one foot on the gas and the other on the brake, so to speak. And we've done that in our dental practices too. This can cause burnout! Leadership is the key to releasing the brakes. Every practice is a result of its' leadership.

You, the leader, set the tone for your practice. Whatever happens throughout your practice is a direct reflection of you and your leadership abilities. Leadership is a privilege...and a responsibility. The responsibility is yours to do what you need to do to become a leader of people.

Why are you in this business? What is your passion? What is your purpose? Do you have a plan? Do you know what steps you will take to fulfill your mission and move in the direction of your vision? Are you in control? These are all questions we will be asking in the next few chapters.

Understand that no one else can build your practice for you until you are willing to take the lead. You don't have to play every position in your practice, but you must understand them. Only then will you be able to lead. When you do you will see an amazing transformation take place in your practice: You won't have to build it alone. Indeed, your team members will gladly and willingly follow your lead and help you build the practice of your dreams. The quarterback position is yours, as well as the cheerleading position. Become a master in these positions and your team members will become the best players you have ever imagined.

Developing leadership skills doesn't come easily or overnight. But those who are willing to work at it and pay the price of learning will have lasting value as the reward. Always remember that becoming a leader isn't a destination you arrive at once and for all. Leadership is an ongoing process. It is a becoming. Without continual training the greatest athlete quickly gets out of shape. Maintaining your leadership position also requires ongoing attention.

> When a leader thinks he or she has learned it all,
> or learned enough, effectiveness begins to diminish.

Here's a quick check-up before we proceed further. Take a few minutes to ask yourself these questions. Jot a few notes down about your responses. With a new understanding of leadership, you might find some areas to work on. Remember, you are the leader of your practice. Do you:

1.   Have a clear vision of the future you want to create?

2.   Remain flexible and open to change?
3.   Identify the needs of your people and then treat them differently, but equal?
4.   Allow yourself and your team members to risk when appropriate and accept mistakes as part of the growth process?
5.   Have clearly communicated high standards and expectations?
6.   Live your life with integrity? Do you *walk your talk?*
7.   Make decisions when needed?
8.   Have a sense of humor...and encourage it in others?
9.   Understand your power and use it wisely?
10. Work to build a team...by being loyal, and by trusting, supporting and serving your employees?
11. Maintain a philosophy of lifelong learning?
12. Consistently model the behavior and attitudes you want from your team?
13. Love yourself, and others, really and truly?

You must finally do the job which is yours alone to do...no matter how much or how little help, encouragement, guidance, instruction and motivation is there along the way. The responsibility is yours to do what you need to do to become a leader of people. Leadership isn't "what you think you are." It is how you are perceived that makes you a leader. Leadership is a privilege and a responsibility. In the end, principled leaders don't have to say anything for us to know who they are...their being says it all.

Right now, ask yourself these two questions:

What have I learned about myself as a leader, so far?

What is one thing I could do as a leader (that I'm not doing now) that if I began today doing it on a regular basis would make a tremendously positive difference in my practice?

Surely the time is now to awaken more fully to our resources. It is a time for new priorities and for disciplining ourselves. And understanding leadership is a key. What is the example you are setting? What kind of leader are you? It's time to make a path, not necessarily follow one. Leaders know that people are more important than things, and they treat them that way. It's time to put the feeling, the compassion, the love...back into leadership. This then, is what the chapters that follow are about. Read them carefully, take them to heart, and employ the principles in your practice. As a result, your workplace will be happier, relationships will be stronger and the fulfillment and satisfaction you feel will be deeper.

Chapter 3

Values

Values are the essence of your practice philosophy. They are the basis of your practice culture. They drive the practice by answering two questions: *(1) What is important to me? and (2) How do we want to act, consistent with our mission, along the path toward achieving our vision?* Values are the deep-seated standards that spread throughout and influence every aspect of the practice: our judgments, our commitments to personal and practice goals, our relationships and communications with others, indeed all our actions and behaviors. Values, essentially, give us our code of conduct. They also provide a source of strength because they give people the power to take action.

It is critical to the practice that the values are clear to each and every person. Every person must know what the practice stands for and be committed to those values. It is our values that provide each team member with a common direction and guidelines for behavior in the practice. Because values run deep, and are emotional, they are often difficult to change. Therefore, it is very important to hire individuals into the practice who already have values in alignment with yours.

Your values are the way you want your practice life (and personal life) to be while pursuing your vision. Where the mission or purpose is very abstract and vision is long term, the values are the daily how to's. They are only helpful, however, if they can be translated into concrete behaviors. You, the leader, must become a master at communicating, promoting, protecting and living out the values of the practice.

Values have to do with being. This must come before the doing and having. If the values are not clear, the doing and having can cause frustration, anxiety, distress, and a host of other uncomfortable feelings *even in the face of seeming success.* And values that aren't in line with the universal principles will not lead us to what we truly desire. The principles will win in the long run, time and time again, because they are the way of the universe. It can be no other way.

Individual intention has an incredible power to fuel your highest aspirations or sabotage your greatest determination, depending upon whether it is focused or fuzzy. If you don't like the results you are getting currently, be willing to take a closer look. Consciously scrutinize your real intentions. Remember as you examine your practice values that you must ask yourself what your personal values are first. These are the core of you as a person. From these will stem the practice values. Once again, if you hold a value to be true personally and try to practice based on something else, you will experience cognitive dissonance which will result in distress, anxiety, frustration and lack of fulfillment...personally and professionally.

We cannot hold one set of values for our dental practice...and hold a different set of values for our personal life. To do so would tear us apart inside. We could not live with separate values split by the time of day. If we say honesty is important, and we value that principle, then that is a value that is a part of our entire life...not just our home life or just our practice life. It is definitely true that we cannot enjoy our vocation, or our life, if we violate our personal values.

It is no surprise that many dentists, and other professionals as well, have very unhappy, unsatisfactory, unhealthy home lives. Where this is the case, often values are not clear, or values that are spoken are not lived out. It is our noble values and truths that keep constant a family. Unfortunately, we are drawn into unhealthy relationships, at times lured in the direction of a grass we believe is greener, only to find ourselves on astroturf. It isn't real. In the process, we tear down what we do have and what is truly important to us. False pride and sex are two causes of disruption, loss and decline in a practice. When we have meaningful values as our guide, and we live out those values, these will not be allowed to become a part of our life and thus a part of our own destruction.

Some examples to get you thinking about values are: trustworthiness, integrity, service, loyalty, honesty, courtesy, commitment, encouragement, ethics, compassion, positive attitude, God, family, sincerity, courage, respect, openness to change, sense of humor, excellence, fidelity, spirituality, and health. The list could go on forever. And here are a few additional ones that relate specifically to your practice: going the extra mile, teamwork, quality, being on time, embracing the diversity of team members, resolving conflict effectively, fun, etc. Begin the process of clarifying your values by asking yourself some questions:

What do you really want in your life?
What do you stand for, personally?
What is truly important to you?
What are your core values and beliefs that will not change?
How do you treat other people?
What does ethical behavior mean to you?
What parts of you are working for you? Against you?
How do *you* define success?
If time, money and other shoulds/oughts/constraints were not present, what would you do?
What are the core values that are more important to you than anything else?
What attitudes and behaviors would mirror these values?
Are you living your life according to what you just identified?

Then continue on and ask yourself these questions about the values of your practice:

Why did you really go into dentistry?
What do you really want in your practice?
What do you really want in the way of production?

What does your practice stand for?
How do you treat your patients (or want to treat them?)
How do you treat your employees?
What does ethical behavior in your practice mean to you?
How do you want to be seen by your patients? By the community?
What attitudes and behaviors in your team members do you want to reward?
What does it mean to act responsibly in the practice?
What attitudes and behaviors, of yourself, would mirror these values?
And with your entire practice team, together ask these questions?
What do we want in our practice?
What do we want in the way of production?
What does the practice stand for?
How do we want to treat our patients?
How do we want to treat each other?
What does ethical behavior mean to us?
How do we want to be seen by our patients? By the community?
What attitudes and behaviors would mirror these values?

Answering these questions might reveal conflicting motivations.....or a conflict between what we say we value and our actual behavior. The principle behind this is: **When what we say we value and the way we actually live our lives is not one and the same, we will experience conflict, distress, tension and reduced results.**

For example, let's say you receive a call from a patient or another doctor and you just don't feel like taking the call so you ask your receptionist to tell the caller you are not in. That's a lie. There are no two ways around it...it just is not the truth.

On the other hand, you say you value honesty, truthfulness and integrity. Your staff hears you make this statement over and over again, but over and over again you ask them to lie for you. This is behavior not in alignment with what you say you value.

Seem trivial? Maybe so at first. But what about the habit pattern it develops? If you ask someone to lie (or you yourself do) in the smallest of things, where does it stop? Your staff now knows that you do not live a life of integrity. *Integrity means walking your talk.* Instead, they see you say one thing and do something else. This unmatched behavior will ultimately cause you distress...that is, if you truly value honesty, truthfulness and integrity. And you will lose respect in the eyes of your team members. They will know the things you say are important really don't mean that much to you.

Although many dentists have reached dramatic results in the levels of productivity they have achieved, for many this "success" hasn't brought the feeling of satisfaction and fulfillment they thought it would. This is a strong indicator that values, or what is truly most important, haven't yet been identified or followed through in action. Becoming clear about your values will help you understand why you are doing what you are doing, not just doing what you do faster and more efficiently.

Are you sincere enough to ask yourself, and others, where your behavior is blocking your desires results?

And, when you identify those barriers, are you willing to acknowledge them and make changes in your thinking and your behavior to lead you to consistency with your professed values?

As we make the personal inventory, there is no need for feeling guilty or placing blame. As we look closely at our lives, both professionally and personally, we might find that we have said certain things are important to us, but we have not been acting in ways consistent with those values. That's okay. In fact, most people, when they first carefully examine their values and behavior, will find that they are not the same. Many people will realize for the first time that they've never taken the time to identify what is truly important to them. They may find they've been motivated by what others think, expect, or do, rather than being internally motivated by what is deeply believed. What is important is that we allow this realization to enlighten us and help us move forward to begin living out what we say is truly important in our lives by aligning our behavior with our values.

> Living out our values will bring us true success,
> satisfaction and fulfillment during our time here on earth.

Abraham Lincoln once said, "I desire to conduct the affairs of this administration that if at the end, when I come to lay down the reins of power, I have lost every other friend on earth, I shall at least have one friend left, and that friend shall be down inside of me."

Values give us the *how* of what we do and the environment in which we practice. They are our internal compass. When we live from our values we keep from burning out. The inner voice that gives rise to our values becomes our constant guide. When we do what we do, personally and professionally, consistent with our values, then we will love what we do. And when what we love to do becomes our priority, our life will be filled with abundance and our satisfaction and fulfillment will increase accordingly.

So many live today in the continual pursuit of more and better...of the secrets of happiness, fulfillment, satisfaction and financial security. A walk through the bookstores will yield hundreds of choices along these subjects, each author having their own remedy or twist to achieve success or mastery in life. But how do you determine it for yourself? It begins by looking within. Take a look at your own true intentions, desires, and your willingness to live them out. Look at the truth of who you are...not who or what other people say you are.

The only way to be happy in dentistry...to be happy in anything...is to be yourself, your best self, and live your life in agreement with that. Those who are happy have learned how to make their practice work in light of their own personal values, and what they want the practice to do and be for them. I believe that's one of the privileges in dentistry. You can build your practice around the real you, allowing you to be yourself and still be a dentist. Although we may look to various things to bring us fulfillment, when we learn that it comes from the inside, we have made our greatest discovery. Change yourself and the way you practice dentistry to fit who you are, and satisfaction will follow...and with that, success.

If you don't like what you're getting back in any area of your life, whether it be your home life, your relationships at the office, your production, your relationships with your patients, whatever it is, examine what you are putting out. What are your thoughts, feelings and actions towards each of these? Our values and our behavior define us. The bottom line is that *we don't get what we want...we get what we are.* Just as we don't change the look of a bedroom by painting the garage, neither will we change our results by changing the outside. We must first make the changes internally.

Read through this next paragraph, then close your eyes and imagine:

Imagine a life of your own design. What is going on? You feel incredibly loved and supported. Your home life is warm and caring, your relationships with your spouse and children are nurturing, loving and committed. The problems you've had now seem to melt away. The walls that were building are beginning to come down. Intimacy has returned. The strong feelings of love are rekindled. You are having fun, enjoying the return home each day.

And what about your practice. What is going on here? You feel wonderful. You've never enjoyed dentistry this much. The person you have had difficulty relating to or communicating with is now highly approachable. The tasks you have met with distaste or hated have actually become fun or interesting. The challenge you were facing has become a success. What is different? See yourself interacting with the patients and with your team members.

Practices today yearn for dentists/leaders who stand for something more than the bottom line. Your values should be the basis for all action in your practice, as well as all policies. Values tell us what we stand for. They give the team members clear direction. Employees need to be guided by values, not so much by rules. When a decision is made on the values you hold dear to your practice, then it is right.

Regardless of what changes occur in the industry, or in the personnel of the practice, or the challenges that occur, the values are what remain unchanged. In the end, the quality of your practice and your life will be a direct result of your values, and the persistence and dedication you give to the commitment of those values.

Chapter 4

MISSION

Knowing what your mission is, then living with and practicing with that purpose is the first step to achieving personal and professional satisfaction.

Your mission *will be* communicated.
If there is none, *that* will be communicated.

Once the values are clear for the practice, the next step is to develop the mission. Your mission or purpose should be the core of your practice. It is not a goal, but a comprehensive guiding direction. Where the values answer the *how,* the mission answers the *why.* **Why do we exist?** Often the mission is not found in the first answer to the why question, but by asking why again and again we often get to the real reason we do our work.

The mission should be greater than for the needs of the employees (a paycheck) or the shareholders (dividends, profits). It should speak to the contribution you make to the community or world in some unique way. It is your distinctive source of value. Excellence requires knowing *what* you do and *why* you do it.

The sense of purpose and togetherness the mission provides helps team members keep their focus and weather the challenges that stand in the way of realizing the vision. With a mission clearly identified and completely accepted by the team, the individuals can be proactive rather than reactive with regard to actions and priorities. It helps the team members make decisions and know what course of action to take. It provides the basis for developing strategy, making choices in resource allocation, and meeting the needs of patients.

The team cannot be expected to deliver the service you want if it isn't defined *and* clearly communicated. Research shows that a person who is highly committed to the mission of the organization is often more satisfied with his or her work than an employee who is less committed, and the committed individual fares much better in times of stress.

Just as with values, before focusing on the practice mission it is important that you take a look at your personal mission. It is difficult to build a meaningful practice without being clear about your personal mission. The mission statement may take the form of a single sentence or several paragraphs. In considering both your personal and practice mission statement, keep in mind that they:

• *Are internal.* Missions come from deep within you; they are not something to impress someone else. It should be something the team takes seriously, feels a part of, and is enthusiastic about carrying out.

• *Speak to your uniqueness...*and what you have to contribute from the "youness" of you.

• *Deal with something greater than you...*with something bigger and higher than yourself. It communicates the actions you need to take to satisfy your patients and keep them happy.

• *Integrate all aspects of you....*spiritual, mental, physical, emotional, and social, and every role you play in your life.

• *Involve at least four areas:* spiritual (the contribution to the practice), psychological (need for growth and development), monetary, and relationships.

- *Are clear, concise and understandable.*

- *Are congruent with your values.* It must be consistent with, built upon, and supportive of the core values, as well as consistent with the practice vision. (See next chapter for vision)

We must not confuse a vision with a mission. The basic mission of a dental practice, upon which to build the balance of the mission statement, will always be to provide dentistry to patients. That hasn't changed. The mission statement, however, should encompass and make very clear how you want your patients to feel. That means things like happy, safe, secure, cared about, comfortable, etc. Many mission statements also refer to the employees. How do they feel? What can they expect? What is the environment? An additional statement on what the employees will give to the practice is sometimes included, such as commitment, extra effort, etc.

Developing Your Personal Mission Statement

To move you into developing your personal mission statement, ask yourself the following questions.

- What do I believe I am capable of?
- Do I love what I do?
- What do I want to be doing?
- What do I want to do now?
- What contributions do I want to make?
- How do I want to be remembered?
- What legacy do I want to leave?
- Professionally, what activities do I feel have the most meaning/greatest worth for me?
- How satisfied am I with my current level of fulfillment in my dental practice?
- What gives my practice meaning?

Without asking these questions it is difficult to put the *doing* part of your practice together in any meaningful way. When we are clear here, we can apply the principles needed to get us where we want to go, and move forward with identifying the *practice* mission statement.

Developing the Practice Mission

- What are you here to accomplish in your practice?
- What is the purpose of your practice?
- What are your practice's strengths and weaknesses? *Consider all areas of your practice, such as attitudes, personalities, talents, operations, etc.*
- Who are your patients?
- What are your patient needs? What problems do they have?
- What do they say they want? What do they say they need?
- How can we enhance those things that bring value to the patient, and change or eliminate those that don't? In other words, what added value do *your* patients receive from your practice that is different from other practices? What makes you unique?
- What are you (and your team) especially good at?

As you begin putting your mission in words, make sure the statement calls forth and stimulates feeling and passion. Understand that a mission statement is more than a slogan. A slogan may focus attention, but it doesn't normally communicate a sense of purpose for the practice. They will not carry the weight or the steadfast power that a mission does. It should say who you are and why you're passionate about it. Focus on the spirit of what you do as you go through this process. Finally, work on it until it becomes so clear that on those difficult days, when you remind yourself of your mission, you redirect your focus and find the strength and optimism of the passion pulling you through. Your mission should be compelling enough that it brings the team together.

The Mission is Never Complete, Once and for All

Take time regularly, perhaps annually, to review your mission. Take your "pulse" not only on where you are headed, but ask yourself if you are continuing to live within the principles you have identified as important. Are you happy with the *becoming* part of you. Are you enjoying the *journey*...and not just trying to reach some destination? Has your mission changed?

Sometimes people are unclear as to which should actually come first, the mission or the vision. Often what happens when the vision is developed before the mission is clear is that the image of the future practice, the vision, becomes impractical because it isn't grounded in what is realistic and based on the specific mission of the organization. There are some occasions, however, for doing this in the reverse order where you really want to move quite drastically into a new arena. In this case it would make sense to work with the vision first, to stretch your imagination and intention. The focus will be broader and less limited by a specific mission.

Finally, ask yourself who should craft your mission statement. Do you want to do it yourself? Or will you involve your team members? If you have a strong team you really enjoy working with and feel you are truly a team working in the same direction, then you will be greatly empowered by having the entire team go through the process. If, however, you are in the position of feeling uncomfortable with your staff and do not feel they are "on board the same ship" you are, then it might be best to do the process yourself, identifying what it is you want your practice to be, and then sharing the mission when complete with your team. If they cannot accept the mission and be committed to it, then perhaps you have a staff member or two who are not the appropriate members for your team and your mission.

Once your mission is clear, the next step is the visioning process. Let's move right along, now, and we'll complete the Values-Vision-Mission process.

Chapter 5

VISION

Where there is no vision, the people perish.
Proverbs 29:18

It is the dentist's responsibility to determine the purpose and philosophy of the practice, and then create the vision that can be shared with the team. Without a clear vision the team is like a ship without a rudder.

The vision answers the question, *What do we want to create?* A vision provides a reference point and a mental model of your practice in the future. It focuses on the longer term orientation and provides a reason for continued growth. It sets the standards of excellence and reflects the high ideals of your practice. A truly powerful vision can make an incredible difference in you, your life, and the lives of your team members.

The process of visioning lays the foundation to break through self imposed barriers about what we have done and how we have done it, and move forward with what we *can* do and *how*. It is about having a sense of what is possible and seeing what others don't necessarily see. It challenges us to look at the practice in new ways. What do we do? Who are our patients? What basic assumptions do we operate from? What internal processes, techniques, systems, and operations reinforce our values? A vision is full of ideas, speculations, desires, assumptions, and certainly value judgments. The vision revisits the values and mission to make sure all three are in alignment.

The greatest inspiration you can provide, as leader, is the power of your conviction. The vision that comes alive is the one you are passionate about. As you see the bigger picture and share it with your team, each person is encouraged and helped to begin thinking more like a leader and moving in the direction of the vision. It helps the team members feel a part of the entire practice, rather than just doing a job that is one piece of the practice. It involves the team in the process of building the practice as a whole.

A clearly communicated vision builds energy and enthusiasm among the team members *because of your passion.* As the energy builds they will begin to feel a sense of responsibility for how the entire team functions...not just for his or her own job. When this occurs, the obstacles, problems, and challenges encountered along the way don't become overwhelming, and are overcome with the passion for the vision. At this point the team will go the extra mile and take extraordinary steps to turn it into reality.

Once people are committed to the vision they will abandon old ways of thinking, old paradigms that get in the way of achieving the vision, and creatively identify exciting new ways to make it happen. With a powerful vision people change. And when people change, things change! A vision, to be effective, must be so strong and have such a powerful pull that you can keep focused on it, and as a result on your goals and objectives, during the good times, as well as the not so good. A vision requires risk taking to get there. But with a clear vision, everyone involved is clear about why they are doing what they are doing in order to make the vision reality.

Let's take it a step further. The vision creates a sense of togetherness, generated by a shared caring of a purpose. *People are connected to it because it reflects their own personal vision.* This is important...it reflects their own personal vision. If a team member's personal vision does not align with your vision for the practice, they will only "sign up" for your's at best. The result will be compliance, not commitment. However, when a team member believes in and commits to the vision it creates a dynamic that touches the core of his or her spirit. It changes your team members relationship to the practice in a most positive way. It ignites enthusiasm and pulls at the heart strings. When people have a common, shared vision, they are more likely to recognize more openly their own personal and professional shortcomings and areas in need of growth.

Developing your Vision

Because the practice is a statement and a tribute to your life, it is important the vision be yours. George Bernard Shaw wrote, "This is the true joy in life, being used for a purpose recognized by yourself as a mighty one." He went on to say, "I am of the opinion that my life belongs to the whole community and as I live it is my privilege—my privilege to do for it whatever I can."

The truly powerful vision contains four elements: (1) it focuses on operations, (2) it includes measurable objectives, (3) it changes the basis for standards in the industry, and (4) it follows from your passion.

A vision is intrinsic...it comes from deep within you. It is the very best of you. It is something you strongly feel, believe and desire. Positive visions come from your aspirations. An extrinsic vision is focusing on achieving something in relation to something on the outside, such as keeping ahead of competition. This is a transitory vision, and once reached the tendency is to go into a protective mode to try and keep it there. An extrinsic vision will weaken the practice over time. If the vision is nothing more than to solve a problem, once the problem is solved the vision is dissolved. Negative visions are those operating out of fear, and fear based visions have very little power. Intrinsic visions, however, have the excitement of building toward something new, better, more dynamic, and purposeful.

Again, your vision should come from your passion, and you do have passion. It is this passion that will direct your vision and mission. It isn't something you have to create out of nothing. It already exists inside you, waiting to be uncovered, identified, brought to the surface and lived out. It may be under so many layers of should's and ought's that the spark seems like it has died. Yet, if you take the time to look inside, you will find it still alive.

What is your vision? Find a quiet, comfortable place to help you clarify your vision and bring it into focus. Allow yourself to invest the time necessary to let the ideas flow, away from interruptions and noise.

Now, allow yourself a few minutes to create a place where you can see your future...where your vision has become reality. Think about some date in the future. Maybe you want to retire from practice at a particular age...perhaps 55 or 60, or maybe 65 or 70. Or maybe you want to focus on a particular year in the future...some ten or twenty years off. Whatever or whenever it is, focus on this time.

Now, see yourself at a celebration in honor of your life...not just of your life as a dentist, but your entire life. Your marriage, your children, your relationships, your employees, your patients...in fact, a celebration of each of your roles. What do you want to see? How does it look? Notice who is there....your immediate family and other relatives, your friends, patients, people you are involved with in organizations and church, your peers, your employees. What do you want these people at your celebration to say? What would you be remembered for? What difference have you made in the world and in the lives of those around you?

Now hold that vision a while longer. Write down what you are seeing. After giving it all the time you need and capturing those images on paper, ask yourself the following questions. Write them down so they become clear and specific. *Remember, the vision is not what the practice is now...it is what you want it to become in the future.*

- What do you want your practice to become?
- If your practice could be anything you wanted in five years, what would it be?
- What is worth your commitment over the next five years?
- What about your practice is unique in the dental field? (How are you different from other practices?)
- What are your practice's opportunities and threats?

Take whatever time you need to pull all your thoughts together and commit them to paper. Your vision needs to be in writing. The only way it will become specific, clear, and able to be thoroughly

communicated is when it is committed to writing. A vision statement may be a few short paragraphs, and it may also be several
pages. Whatever it takes for you to develop your vision fully is
how long it should be.

As you determine your vision, remember that the only way to
be happy and fulfilled in dentistry (or anything else in life) is to be
yourself, and be your best self. Don't try to become someone else.
That doesn't mean that you don't grow and progress, but it does
mean that you don't do something just because somebody else
does it or to keep up with the dentist next door.

> A vision that is not consistent with values
> will fail to inspire or motivate, and may
> actually create or engender cynicism.

Any changes you make should be changes of choice so you can
practice dentistry that is consistent with your passion and your
values. No one can be truly happy or sincerely enjoy their vocation, regardless of what it is, if they violate personal values.

> Although we may look to various outside factors to
> bring us fulfillment, when we learn that it comes
> from the inside, we have made our greatest discovery.

Make sure you practice dentistry and live your life so you don't
compromise your values. Satisfaction will follow, and with it success, *your style*, following right on its heels. Quality in dentistry is
related to the fulfillment of your purpose, to the lives that you
touch...and one of the most important is yours!

Gaining Acceptance and Commitment From the Team

Developing a shared acceptance and commitment to vision begins
with communicating your vision to your team members, as well
as discussing how each has a role in making the vision a reality.
This involves:

•   Clearly expressing the vision so it is understood. Include
your philosophyand beliefs that support the vision, as well as rea-

sons for the practice's existence and aspirations for the future.

• Why the vision is needed and why it is important to the practice. Communicate relevance. Why is this direction important? This may involve sharing strategic information with your team members so they can better understand. Individuals operating in ignorance mistrust, lack commitment, resist change, and question motives.

• Why the vision is important to each team member. How does it relate to the work they each perform. How does what they do play a part in realizing the vision? Be sure to allow immediate opportunities for them to act on it. Enthusiasm is dampened rapidly if there is no outlet for them to act on a new vision.

• What areas can we work on now? Are there areas where behavior needs to be changed? Attitudes? And then provide any necessary mechanisms for that change.

• Finally, your commitment. State it verbally, then back it up with action. Your team members need to feel and sense your passion for the vision. Belief in your vision and integrity of leadership (acting in a manner consistent with your vision and values) is vitally important in order to motivate your employees, and gain their trust and respect.

Put your vision in writing...consider every word. It may take one page, it may take five. Whatever it takes, invest the time necessary to put in writing the vision you have for your practice. Then have the team members read it. Get the team to talking about it. Discuss it. Brainstorm what it will take to get there and build to the expected commitment from each staff member. Once you have agreement, then reward and recognize behavior that is consistent with what it will take to make the vision reality.

The key to the effectiveness of your vision will be having the entire team accept the vision. This may mean a paradigm shift about what is important for them and the practice. This is critically important because *unless they feel they have chosen* to adapt to new paradigms, practices and methods, the tendency will be to revert to old ways. The challenge is to overcome the resistance to change in order to maintain the status quo. With vision, a powerful vision, there is no room for status quo.

As a leader you must be open to knowing yourself, as well as your team members. You need to know where they are, where they want to go, the progress they have made, and where each team member stands in relation to the practice and its' vision. It takes *knowing*. Guessing, estimating, thinking and assuming aren't enough. You may find in the process that you have a team member or two who is not on board with the vision, and who has no intention of changing. When this is the situation, a caring discussion with that employee will be necessary to determine what the future of that employee is. As you hire new employees, hire people who have a belief system and values consistent with yours.

Building on the vision takes teamwork, change within the organization and communication. It cannot and will not happen with everyone doing their own thing without regard for the other. It will not happen if you have employees who are interested solely in their paycheck.

The Values, Vision and Mission Model

The Principled Practice will operate smoothly because the vision, values and mission are clearly defined, articulated and accepted by the entire team. Look at the model below. Having these clearly identified makes handling the day to day process of the practice quite simple.

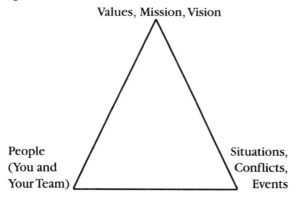

Values, Mission, Vision

People
(You and
Your Team)

Situations,
Conflicts,
Events

Notice the left corner of the triangle: People.And notice the right corner of the triangle: Practice policies, structures, situations, events, conflicts, problems, etc.

When the vision, mission and values are clear, regardless of the circumstances or problems...whatever comes up in the practice...you simply assess the situation in light of the values, mission and vision, and then decide how you will respond to the situation. The same goes for policies and procedures. When you are establishing new policies, be sure to run them past your values, mission and vision to make sure they are consistent. The beauty of the triangle model is that it is no longer necessary to banter back and forth between the people side and the situation side. When this happens it is often difficult to gain clarity on how to best handle the situation. Worse yet, you may find yourself running in circles with a conflict or problem, or perhaps not doing anything, because you are unsure. With the values, mission and vision as your guide you can evaluate any situation much more clearly, quickly and effectively. Your values, mission and vision give you a guiding light....the lighthouse in the storm, the candle in the darkness to show you the way.

Is Your Vision Working?

If you think you have a vision that is effectively driving the practice, here is a quick test to see if it measures up. Ask yourself these questions:

• Can you put your finger on the vision? Is it clearly stated and does *everyone* in practice know what it is? Can your team members verbalize it?

• Does it include what it is you do, who you serve, your desired level of quality and efficiency, how you respond, issues of professionalism, etc.?

• Does the vision statement include all areas of the practice?

• If your practice continues on its present course, five or ten years down the road will you be closer to your vision? If not, where are you headed?

• Does everything in your practice, from processes, information systems, operational systems, methods, incentives and everyone (you and every member of your team) support the vision and back it up with actions, attitudes and behaviors?

• Are you consistently moving in the direction of your vision? Are *all* team members committed to the vision and doing their part in taking action to achieve the vision?

• Are you open to and making changes necessary to insure that you continue to progress toward your vision?

• Are your goals and priorities in line with your vision? Are you monitoring them regularly to insure they are in line?

• Do your patients look favorably on the direction your practice is headed?

• How do you know? How are you doing in the patient relations area?

• Have new threats or opportunities arisen in the marketplace that affect your vision? If so, have you addressed them and are you working on ways to make necessary changes?

Remember, having a clearly articulated vision is important to you, but it is also important to the rest of the team. They want to know where the practice is headed. They feel much better about their work when there is a compelling vision they are working toward. It may be very clear to you what it takes for your patients to give you the very best rating, but until every team member is involved and truly understands the vision, it won't happen.

A dental practice, to succeed, thrive and grow in the future, must be led by a visionary leader. Driven by patient demands and rapid technological change, we must stay ahead by remaining in an open position of continually asking questions. Visionary leaders, rather than being problem solvers when problems arise (expected or unexpected), must be problem finders. They will look down the road to what is ahead. The rapid pace at which we are moving is much like driving a high speed vehicle. If you wait until you see something *clearly* in the road ahead before you consider what move to make, it may be too late. Accordingly, in our practices, we must not wait until we see completely clearly before we begin to consider the possibilities and ramifications, the challenges and the opportunities. If we do wait we will find that we have been rolled over by a freight train traveling at full steam ahead, or we will find ourselves wondering why the great opportunities pass us by. We must move before challenges or possibilities appear right on our doorstep; waiting may mean "too late."

Because we live in a dynamic world, our vision must be dynamic, not static. As you travel further down the road, your vision may take on a different characteristic, and that's perfectly okay. In fact, the vision should be revisited on a regular basis (perhaps annually) to make sure it is still in line with your thinking and aspirations. Your vision is a part of the ongoing process of keeping your practice up-to-date and integrated with the changes in the outside world as constant new realities emerge.

It is with our values, vision and mission as our blueprint that we can stand strong in the face of change. It is having a changeless core of values on the inside that allows us the freedom and ability to change in these times of rapid transformation. When these are not clear, and the winds of change blow strong, we find ourselves grasping for our next move.

There is no big step to success. It is one small step in the right direction, followed by the next and then the next. That will get you to where you want to go...as long as your direction is clearly identified.

Successful dental practices aren't more successful than others simply because the team members have greater clinical skills or more opportunities than others. Instead, they are successful because they have direction: the leader has a clear vision and focus, and has learned how to apply the basics of effective leadership and important principles to gain the enthusiasm and commitment of the team to work toward that vision.

It takes clarity of all three...vision, values and mission...to feel comfortable and confident. Without any one of them, we will continually compare ourselves to others. We will try to determine how "good" we are by seeing how we "measure up" to those around us. When we do this we are driving ourselves into frustrating territory where we feel out of control.

> All we can really deal with is our own potential,
> and determine what is important to us.

When we do, we can live in peace and harmony, feeling satisfied with the meaning of our life.

Chapter 6

GOALS

Once your vision, values, and mission are clearly established, written, and the entire team is on board, take the time to identify your goals. Where the vision is the picture of the future you would like to see, goals are the means of getting there. Nothing becomes dynamic until it first becomes specific. Goals help you bring the vision, values and mission to life on a daily basis. They give direction and help you determine what your daily activities must be in order to reach those goals, and move forward in your mission and vision.

The process of setting goals, making decisions, and implementing actions guided by the spirit of service and commitment to values is essential to the realization of the higher standard of leadership that is so important in our practices today. If we don't know what we stand for, what is important to us, what our purpose is, then it is difficult to set goals that are meaningful, let alone achieve them. Therefore, goals must be consistent with your values, mission and vision.

Goals are important for each member of your team. And, involving the entire team in establishing practice goals gives them the much needed and desired feeling of belonging. To begin, get your team together and share your individual goals. You take the lead. Be the model and share with them your one year, five year, ten year, even lifetime goals. Then have them share theirs. Something amazing happens when we do this. Team members begin to understand their doctor better and when this happens an amazing change begins to take place. They begin to see you as a real person.

As you begin the process of clarifying and establishing practice goals, ask what is necessary. As a team, ask yourself these questions:

• What needs to change in order for our behavior, our actions, to be consistent with our mission, vision and values.

• What needs to change in our attitudes for them to be consistent with our mission, vision, and values?

• What do we need to do differently in relation to our interaction with patients? With each other?

• What is the value of each patient?

Then ask these questions that will lead you closer to your strategic goals.

• What are the key quantitative indicators (numbers) that measure our success? (Production, collections, average daily production, number of referrals, case acceptance percentage, percentage of preappointed hygiene appointments, number of days missed by employees, patient satisfaction, etc.)

• What are our unique factors? What differentiates us?

• What is our perceived value by our patients? What do our patients expect from us?

• What can we do to meet their needs more effectively than we have in the past?

Your dental practice is like a prism, reflecting rays of whatever is present. There are so many facets of the practice, each adding to the spectrum as a whole. Here are some measures of the prism that must be considered as you set your goals and develop your action plan:

Profitability Factor: These include all the overhead costs (such as office supplies, dental supplies, lease or mortgage, equipment, lab, salaries, continuing education, etc.)

Relationship Factor: This includes the patient relations or customer service perception. What is your patients' perception of your quality and value? What is your image and reputation? How efficient and prompt are you (on-time)? Do your patients feel they receive high value at a reasonable cost?

Innovative Factor: How innovative are you and your staff? Do you maintain state-of-the-art equipment and materials? How often do you involve yourself and your staff in continuing education (clinical, materials, personal growth...all aspects of the business)? How often do you, your staff and your patients come up with new ideas or suggestions? Are you asking your staff and patients for input?

Staff Factors: Is your workplace safe, clean and up to standards (yours and OSHA's)? Do you have frequent employee turnover? Do you do ongoing training? Are you providing your employees with the necessary tools to do the job well? Do your employees feel appreciated? Do you really have a team (not just a group)? Is there integrity of all staff members?

Market Factors: These are factors affecting your growth, involving increased production, market share, retention of patients, flow of new patients and visibility of practice.

Characteristics of Goals

It is helpful to understand the characteristics of goals as you prepare for the goal setting process. Each goal should be:

Personal. This means you own your goal. If it doesn't come from inside you, it will be difficult to achieve.

Positively stated. I will...not *I will not.* The mind cannot picture a void.

Specific. State your goal clearly and specifically.

Measurable. If your goals are not measurable, you will not be able to check your progress, and you will not know when you have reached it.

Time targeted. If there is no date for achievement, your goals will keep marching ahead into the future, just as you do, without being achieved.

Big, but realistic. If they are not big there will be nothing to generate enthusiasm. If it is too big or unrealistic one of two things can happen: (1) it will not generate enthusiasm because it seems unreachable, or (2) if it is missed by a wide margin it can have a psychological impact for future accomplishments in a negative way.

Consistent with your values, other goals and circumstances. Make sure you are not establishing conflicting goals. This leads to internal conflict, frustration, stress, and cognitive dissonance.

Long range. It is necessary to set goals far enough out so you are not stumped by short term roadblocks and obstacles.

Daily. Goals need to be worked on daily in order to move continually forward toward their achievement. Specified activities on a daily basis are important.

Written. If they aren't written, they probably won't happen.

Worthy of your commitment. If not, then you better reevaluate because they probably won't happen!

Finally, we can move into the actual strategic goals by asking the question: *What do we want to achieve in the next year?*

This is where you make *decisions* and become *specific* about where you will focus your energy and efforts in the next year. When we set goals personally, to remain in balance we must consider every area of our lives. The same is true of our practice. We need to consider every area of the practice when we establish our goals. This could be anything from increased new patient flow, greater treatment acceptance, focusing on a particular niche or narrow market focus, building relationships in the office, working on teamwork...you name it. The key here is to be very clear about your focus and be committed to staying with this focus even when the going gets tough.

> Nothing becomes dynamic until
> it first becomes specific.

That means we must be focused, believe, and have a clear vision of whatever it is we want. We must visualize it already completed.

Determine Your Priorities

After you have identified the goals you wish to achieve, it is important to establish priorities. Sometimes we have too many goals to work on at once...or we have some longer range goals that really can't be accomplished unless a shorter range goal is completed. Prioritizing helps eliminate conflicting goals too. Prioritize to determine what is most important right now. This clarifies and helps us gain proper perspective and focus.

An easy way to prioritize is to list every goal on a flip chart or black board. Then, begin by comparing the first goal listed to every other goal. Read the second goal and ask "Which is more important at this time...the first or the second?" Then make a mark by the one identified. Then read the first against the third asking the same question. Again, make a mark next to the priority goal. Read the first goal against every other goal, marking the priority, until you have the first goal compared to every other goal. Then begin the process again beginning with the second goal. Read the second goal against the third, fourth, fifth, etc. Complete this process until you have compared every goal against the other. When completed, count the number of marks you have by each goal and put them in order of importance based on your marks.

This is an easy way to identify what really is the most important to you. Often what happens is that a person finds out the goal that has been floating around in their mind for a couple years, but has never been accomplished, just wasn't as important as something else. Understand, however, that just because a goal ranks at the bottom doesn't mean it isn't important. It just means that it isn't as important *at this time* as something else.

Action Plans

Once you have identified and prioritized your goals, it's time to define the action plan needed to turn them into reality. Activities are what we do daily to reach our goals. They should always be planned with the bigger picture in mind. These activities should be in line with our mission and values, and move us closer to our vision each day. Each goal should be put through the same process of identifying the activities necessary to reach the goal.

Sometimes it is difficult to come up with ideas for how you can get to where you want to go. This is where involvement by the entire team is incredibly beneficial. Begin the brainstorming process by asking these questions of every goal you have established:

What are all the activities we can think of that can lead us to our goal?

What else will it take to reach this goal? That is, what might we need to change in order to achieve this goal?

Brainstorming with your staff on the action steps is helpful. Before saying yes or no to any ideas, write them all on a flip chart. Realize that no idea is bad. Without judgment, brainstorm as many different ways as you can to get to where you want to go. Once you have exhausted the possibilities...then go back and discuss what, out of the entire list, fits in with your values, mission and vision. Then ask yourselves if you are committed to making this happen? It makes no sense to establish an action plan to which no one is committed. The most successful people, in any field, are those that take action. They are those who have a vision of what they want to be and who have the persistence to keep taking action in line with that vision even when the going gets tough. Remember: Vision without action is only dreaming.

Review Your Goals Regularly

Review your goals regularly to determine whether or not you are on course, or if your course needs correction. If you have veered off the course ask the question "Why?" Perhaps you find the path you took is not leading where you expected. As a team, brainstorm what needs to happen to get you back on the path headed in the direction of your choice. Determine for yourself how often you want to formally make the review, but do it at least annually. The tremendous changes in dentistry today would suggest that perhaps a more frequent examination would be appropriate, to insure you are moving forward in the direction you choose.

Follow Your Heart

It is important to realize in all this discussion about vision, mission, values, goals, etc. that we must follow our heart. Sometimes that means clearing out a lot of old "stuff" so we don't keep repeating old stories over and over. So many people today are rushing in so many different directions, not sure just exactly what they want or are looking for, not sure why they are doing what they are doing, not really sure about much at all. It's time to slow down. Listen to that voice inside and be still. We each must realize that if the "thing" at the end of the journey is what we're after, we'll be disappointed when we get there. It will never really be what we thought. We must enjoy the journey along the way.

We all choose our own experiences by the actions we take and nothing happens by accident. The principle or universal law of cause and effect is always in place and affects everything we do. To be human means to take responsibility for one's life and for the consequences of our actions. Does that mean we will always be successful? That depends upon our definition of success. When we experience failure, if we look at it for what it is, we can grow tremendously and move forward in the direction of our dreams.

Failure only tells us that we have another opportunity to grow. It is a stepping stone to something greater if we will but open our eyes to the lesson inherent in the situation.

Do we always reach our goals? Yes. We always reach our goals according to our concepts, our values and our beliefs. In fact, our beliefs (spiritual, physical, emotional, and mental) are the currency with which we achieve our goals. We believe and achieve according to our level of value. The problem is that so many people don't live their values, often because they don't know what those values are. They haven't taken the time to ask themselves the question.

If you don't like the results you are getting, take a look at your belief system. You prove what you believe by your results. For example, the person who continues to enjoy a failure experience has a stronger belief in failure than in success. Belief dictates results! Perhaps you have believed there just aren't enough good employees these days. Most likely, you are living that out in your results as well. You don't have the staff you would like to have. Perhaps you're feeling that there just aren't enough patients out there either. If that's what you truly believe, that's what you'll attract as well. The beautiful part is that our beliefs are our evaluation of something, and we are free to change our evaluation of anything!

Unfortunately our mind's natural negative alignment tends to make us think that our miracles, goals, plans, and dreams are not going to come true. By virtue of the programming we have experienced throughout our lives, many have a deep down belief that they really won't achieve what they would like to achieve. We must remember that our potential is limited to what is logical to ourselves. This is true for each of us...and for each of you in your practice team. And, what we don't believe, we won't achieve.

Results come from habits, and habits come from attitudes. Look at any result in your life and you can tell where it came from. Motivation begins it...discipline completes it.

Getting Off the Treadmill

"I set goals, but I never seem to follow through." If this is your situation, you must realize that until you get off the treadmill and get started you will never achieve your goal. Wishing won't make it come true. If you are having this problem, ask yourself:

- Is this *my* goal? Or am I living out someone else's should's?
- Have I crystallized and focused my thinking?
- Have I put together an action plan to achieve my goal...with a time target?
- Do I have confidence in myself and my ability to succeed?
- Do I believe I am worthy of success?
- Do I have the unceasing determination to do what it takes, regardless of the obstacles I meet?
- Is the goal really worth it to me?
- Am I aware of and working with the universal principles to my benefit?

Until you have answered yes to each of these questions, you will most likely find it difficult to move forward on a consistent basis with your action plan.

What About the Obstacles?

There will always be obstacles. The question really is, "When I meet them, how will I handle them?" The biggest trouble maker for most people is that they imagine problems and quit before they get started, or begin the project half-heartedly. Remember, problems are inventions of the mind, they are perceptions we have.

We were never promised a paved road to success; not even a smooth one! In fact, if we find ourselves on a paved road we'll probably find it isn't the one leading us where we want to go. The road to success is always under construction. The road to our own personal and professional growth is always under construction. We are, throughout our life, always under construction!

> Circumstances color the picture...but your attitude
> determines the shade.

It is not what happens to you that is so important (circumstances), rather what you do with them is what is important.

An Ongoing Process

The enjoyment we experience from the goals we attain is in direct proportion to the enjoyment we have while reaching, striving and working toward them. It is the journey that counts. It is what we become as we work towards our goals that is important. It is the process.

Remember these few principles as you set about your goals and action plan:

- For conditions to change, for your practice or your life to change, you must change.
- Concentrate on what you want, not on what you don't want. Whatever you focus on you will draw to you.
- You can have anything you want when you develop the consciousness to receive it.

As we end this chapter...take a few minutes to reflect on the following.

Project yourself into the future and your practice. If you stay on the course you are on now, will you like the result five years from now? If not, what are you willing to do differently today to produce different results tomorrow?

Remember, the place you will spend the rest of your life, personally and professionally, is being created right now, today. Your daily accomplishments are the bricks building the stairway to wherever it is you want to go.

Chapter 7

PERSONAL

Are you making time for your family? Do you have fun to-gether? Are you really communicating? Has the intimacy disap-peared from your family and marriage relationship? Although you communicate for a living, what is happening at home? Would your family say of you, "You don't know how to communicate."

Although this is a book about your practice, it would not be complete without considering the personal and spiritual dimen-sion of your life. It is from this aspect of our being that meaning and purpose is made known. Our life is not separated neatly into different pieces in time. Time has long since passed when we could look at our lives and separate them into segments...this is my per-sonal, this is my professional, this is my social, etc. Nor can we separate the parts by applying different values or principles to each. In other words, it is not possible to live one set of values at the office, and another set of values when you are "off duty." Attempt-ing to live in this manner causes conflict, frustration, anxiety, and distress, not to speak of troubled relationships.

What many are missing in their lives, no matter how much they have, is a sense of meaning. Many are feeling the unrest of accomplishment without meaning, of acquisition without satisfaction, of running to the next stop without understanding the destination. What about you? Are you on this same path, running the same race? This is a spiritual question because it is about ultimate values and ultimate concerns. The need for meaning is not biological and not psychological, but spiritual.

Our society has developed in such a manner that we have placed magnified importance on the material aspects of our existence. Many are continually chasing after more, better, bigger, faster, newer, quickest, greatest...you name it. Certainly most of us in dentistry enjoy the luxuries and comforts of life we have come to call necessity, but where do we say enough? We become so involved with the *doing* and *having* that sometimes we miss the *being*. Chasing after the next item on our list of acquisitions, we seldom stop and ask the question, "How will I know when I have enough? And then what will I do?"

> Nothing gives so much direction to a person's
> life as a sound set of values.
> *Ralph Waldo Emerson*

Let's go back to values. When you were examining your values as they relate to the practice, did you also ask yourself what you value personally? If not, it's time to look within and examine the contents. Values are the foundation of our character. And we are responsible for our character...not God, not mom or dad, not the church, the state, or the government. Values are clearly tied to purpose. If we don't know what we stand for, what is important, we will find it difficult in the face of varying circumstances to confidently make a decision as to our behavior and actions. It is also difficult to set goals that are meaningful without clearly understanding our values.

What is important to me?
What do I want to become?
Am I operating out of someone else's values?
What is the purpose of my family?
What is the purpose of my marriage or significant other relationship?

It is equally important to establish goals, to have a vision and mission for yourself personally and for your marriage, as it is for your practice. They need to be developed by you, individually, as well as with your spouse. When you take the time to work through and discuss these, you can then check to make sure they are not in conflict. If they are, further discussion and communication is needed.

Every area of your life is important to examine when you are setting goals in order to remain balanced. Here are a few areas to consider: personal development, children, marriage, social, health, spiritual, physical, intellectual, recreational, financial, community, and vocational.

Sometimes it takes a wake-up call to make us stop long enough to ask these questions and determine the direction in which we are headed. A friend of mine received a wake-up call in the form of breast cancer five years ago. Four years later her husband, in a routine blood test, was found to have leukemia. Another colleague was recently diagnosed with multiple sclerosis. Another was served with divorce papers. Many people in California experienced a great deal of loss because of the massive January 1994 earthquake. In other parts of the country people have lost everything they own in floods. Will it take that for you? And did it do the job for them? Or are these people still running after the *doing* and *having*, forgetting about the most important question...who am I *becoming*. What about you, have you learned to *be*? Let's look at a few additional examples.

Tom says his family is important to him. He really wants to maintain a close family relationship. He values time with his children and his spouse. But Tom's behavior looks totally different. Tom spends increasing hours at the office, can't seem to make it to his children's soccer games or back-to-school nights because of golf, meetings, you name it. Something always comes up. He seems to forget that his children won't be young forever; they won't live at home forever; he will not have the opportunity to watch them grow, participate in events that are meaningful to them, and attend soccer games forever.

Patricia is not married. She does say, however, that she values time with her friends. But Patricia hasn't seen many of her friends for months. "There's never enough time," she says as she's off on business running around the country, more concerned with how high she can build her bank account. She's obsessed with more, bigger and better. But when it comes to her friends, what she says is important isn't happening. As a result, Patricia has become a very lonely woman, destined to share her evenings with four hotel walls and dining out alone.

Jerry is married. Jerry says he values his relationship with his wife. He even says he loves her. But those that work with Jerry in the practice know that he is having an affair with one of his employees. Behavior and values matched? Not even close.

These are but a few examples of behaviors and values that are not in alignment. Again, the net result is conflict, distress, disharmony, anxiety and a host of other negative feelings.

Tom will reap a negative reward one of these days. He will wake up and find that he doesn't know his children, he wasn't a part of their growing up, and he can never get that back. It may even be that Tom's children will become so busy, taking after their Dad's example, that *they* won't have time for *him*. Patricia may reap a negative reward too. She might wake up years from now realizing that she never even lived! She spent a whole lot of time working, earning money, and accumulating material goods, but nothing of importance or lasting value was achieved. And Jerry? Well, Jerry may have a rude awakening one day when he finds that his wife has left him...and he has nothing left of a relationship he once said was so important.

An article in the ADA News told the story of four boys who sat around the fire after a cookout and played the wish game. Each told what they wished for the most. One boy wanted to be a second baseman for the Atlanta Braves, another wanted a car, and another wanted to be a policemen. The final boy, however, *wished that his daddy loved him more than his beeper.*

Why do we do this to ourselves and to our families? Is it because we don't know any better? Or because we simply haven't asked ourselves the values questions and established our priorities? Either way, it is important to realize that every single minute we are alive we are trading that moment of life for something in return. Can you honestly say you are happy with the trade? Is it meaningful? Are you so busy accomplishing and accumulating that you are missing out on living?

If you are not happy now,
you will not be any happier with "more" of anything.

The foundation of our lives needs to be secure, and that requires having the *right priorities*. Norm and I share the same foundation, the same priorities. First, God; second, family; and third, business. Are you clear on your values...or will it take a wake-up call to force you to take a look? When we are not sure about our values temptation creeps into our lives through many doors. And it is the inability or unwillingness to resist temptation that often gets us into trouble or on some distant path leading us in a direction away from our dreams, beliefs and values. If we are determined to resist temptation we must do four things:

• We must not be weakened by situations. This means we must not give in to circumstances or situations that compromise us, our values, our integrity.

• We must not be deceived by the persuasive attempts of others or situations to pull us off course.

• We must not be gentle with our emotions. Sometimes we must pull ourselves back to our principles and values and forego an emotional pull toward an unhealthy, compromising situation.

• We must not be confused with something that can give immediate results, gratification, pleasure, etc. that is *for the moment* and pulls us away from our values.

These are principles we must live by in our personal and professional lives if we are to live with harmony, peace, fulfillment, joy, and integrity. We will never truly enjoy our vocations if we violate our personal values in the process. Those of us who want to keep our garden healthy and hearty must not reserve a plot for the weeds. We must plant the strong, healthy principles of love, honesty, truth, commitment, fidelity, selfless giving, consideration, and compassion. These principles, when lived out, provide for a strong, healthy, meaningful marriage that creates transformed partners. Where principles of evil, dishonesty, and infidelity exist, we are drawn away from love and our resistance deepens to all that is good in our relationship. Most of us would agree that we want the benefits a healthy marriage brings, but are we willing to make the commitment it takes? Are we willing to apply these principles and *live them out* on a day by day basis, renewing our commitment to them each day? Fail at love and the rest doesn't matter.

So seldom in our marriage relationships, or long-term relationships with significant others, do we talk about what we appreciate in that person. Yet without this the relationship will suffer and certainly not give the pleasure and fulfillment it could otherwise. Perhaps it is time to make the time to rediscover what you really value in your mate.

Danny Thomas has said, "In an effort to insure my children's tomorrows, I have lost their todays." What about our children? We want the benefits of healthy relationships with our children, but are we willing to make the commitment to the time and energy it takes to love and to nurture, to educate and train, to listen and respond?

As we look at our home lives, we must remember that no success in practice will ever make up for failure at home. Just as it is important for your dental practice to continually change and grow to survive and thrive, it is important that your marriage and family relationships grow and expand. The alternative is to find it broken and in need of repair, and possibly beyond repair in the mind of one of the individuals involved.

Many dentists, if not most, are in an enviable position according to much of our population. Others see dentists as having plenty, of having the "good life." But having a substantial amount of money can actually keep us insulated and isolated, thinking we don't need much, and certainly not connected. But when problems surface, boredom strikes, or when a wake-up call hits, that's when the isolation turns to feelings of pain, friendlessness and insecurity...regardless of the bottom line on the financial statement.

The problem we face is a spiritual one. It is not one of money, of having enough, of doing enough. It comes from the inside. It has to do with meaning, with being. It has to do with the love question. Ram Dass puts it well, "We are not human beings having a spiritual experience. We are spiritual beings having a human experience." Many of us have tried to separate the spiritual from our everyday living, which is much of the problem. We have left unattended that which is there for us every moment of every day. For many, the spiritual is connected with church services, meditation, yoga, a trip to Peru or India, praying, reading religious literature, etc. We think these things are more spiritual than taking a walk, riding a bike, preparing dinner, playing with your canine companion, talking with your spouse, making love, helping your child with his homework, talking with your dental staff, or working on a patient. We try to separate the spiritual from the everyday and wonder why we feel a sense of meaninglessness, devoid of purpose and fulfillment.

Spirituality has to do with *oneness* and *wholeness*. That means putting our life back together and opening ourselves to finding the spiritual within the ordinary and everyday experiences of our lives. There's nothing else we really need...nothing else to acquire...nothing else to get or do to bring us back to wholeness. We already have everything we need.

When we awaken to the wholeness of who we are; when we take the time to develop our vision, mission and values and then strategically plan and set goals; and when we are willing to maintain a balance in our lives of all that we do, we will find a new level of satisfaction, fulfilllment and success.

It is there for every one of us, if we will but live out the principles of integrity, responsibility, trust, discipline and balance. We can have most everything we want in life if we will work for it. For many, however, it comes as a big realization that what we really need to work toward is not just the productivity in our practices to have more money...but we need to work on the *inner* part of us, the *being* part. We need to get clear about what we really want, about what is really important to us, and then live by the principles that will assure we are headed in the right direction. Then, and only then, will we know true success. Then, and only then, will we know the thrill, the satisfaction and the fulfillment of life at it's best, personally and professionally.

Part Two

*You and Your Employees:
Building Your Team*

Chapter 8

Before You Hire: Develop Your Plan

There is no such thing as a self made person. We all need others to achieve and grow, as well as to recover from disaster or adversity. We are absolutely powerless unless we are willing to say, "I need help." Think about it....regardless of what our goals are in dentistry, we are dependent upon others for our success. Without our patients we could achieve nothing; without our suppliers we would have nothing with which to work; and without our employees, practicing dentistry would be very difficult at best. In dentistry, we must share the vision...and ask for help.

Success can never be achieved alone.

When we talk about expenses of a practice, we include the salaries of our staff. We look at them as overhead, which they are, but they are much more important than simply being overhead. They are an *investment* we make to return great dividends. Return on investment doesn't simply mean productivity results. It means the people and service factor, and in the long run the fulfillment factor.

The very nature of our business gives us a key to success. Health care is a vocation based on service and commitment to helping people. This requires that we have the right people with the right characteristics to provide health care services that feel right and good to the patients. People are the key to this success. We need people who are caring and compassionate, who will listen to patients and understand what they are saying, as well as what they are unable to articulate but want to communicate.

If we ever hope to get things right on the outside (with our patients), we must first work to get them right on the inside (with our team). Although changes meet us at every front in dentistry today, one of the greatest concerns for dentistry in the new millennium is the hiring, retention and development of the professional team. Your practice is really only as good as....no, not just you...but your employees.

Poor selection in the hiring process costs valuable time and money, requires increased energy and counseling time, reduces productivity, and creates low morale. Applicants who may be impressive during an interview may prove to be a hiring mistake later if the process is not well defined.

Given the significant cost of poor hiring decisions, it is important to *increase interviewing effectiveness*. To do this, careful attention must be given to each phase: planning the interviews, conducting the interviews, evaluating the applicants, and making the hiring decision.

Overview of the Hiring Process

You must commit yourself to hiring only those people you respect and with whom you believe you will enjoy working. It is important to consider the image they will give your practice, because patients judge a practice by the team the doctor has chosen. Hiring decisions made too quickly can and will affect your practice, how people perceive your practice, and ultimately your bottom line. It certainly will make a difference in how the team functions as a team. For this reason, skimping in the interviewing process is being penny wise and pound foolish.

Take the time to interview enough people so you select from a "pool" of good candidates. Hire people who are motivated and enthusiastic; people who want to help you build a practice that stands out, that *makes* a difference...that *is* different. If you really want this kind of practice you must begin with people who feel that way themselves and who are willing and able to make that difference a reality. You won't find these individuals in the bottom of the barrel of the hiring reservoir; nor will you find them among the people who are willing to settle for the lowest salary levels.

Too often what passes for the interview and selection process is nothing more than a newspaper ad, and an employee chosen from whatever candidates emerge...*whether or not any of them actually fit your profile and are the kind of person you really want to employ.* Employee selection is critical. Because of this, it is important to select only when you find the person you feel is *really* right for *your* practice.

Recently in our practice we went through a five month period of using temporary hygienists while we continued our search for the hygienist who would best serve and be served by our practice. Working with temporary hygienists wasn't the ideal situation, but it was the best choice for the bigger picture. When patients asked what was going on we told them enthusiastically, "We're looking for just the right individual to become an integral part of our team. We want someone who will give you and all our patients the exceptional service you deserve and have come to expect from our practice." When we finally found Tami, we knew that our search efforts, patience and persistence had paid off. She is one in a million.

What is needed in the dental practice are strong and effective team members who are both leaders *and* followers. An effective team member is a person who is a self-starter, thinks for herself, and carries out her responsibilities with enthusiasm and passion. This person is a risk taker and an independent problem solver, and as such builds competence and focuses efforts for the greatest results. Additionally, this person can manage herself well and is courageous, credible, honest, and trustworthy. She has made a commitment to the practice and to the purpose, principles, and mission that stand at the center of the practice. It is important to understand that this strong employee will often see herself as an equal to the leader, except in terms of responsibilities. She is well-balanced and responsible. She can succeed without strong leadership, but will blossom even more with a quality leader. Surrounded by these types of team members, the dentist's leadership position is made much easier.

Although it takes time and effort to recruit, interview, and hire quality individuals, it is time and energy well invested. These strong individuals give the practice a significant financial advantage because they eliminate much of the need for elaborate supervisory systems. They will be responsible for carrying through their responsibilities, will make good use of their time so hours are not wasted, and you'll get maximum results for the time invested.

Further, other team members, as well as the dentist, like working with these individuals because their hearts are in their work. Morale is high, and energies and loyalties are channeled for the good of the practice. These people will look for ways to grow, for training and development, rather than expecting it to come to them. They won't have to be force-fed. In short, these individuals have the overall picture as well as the detail; the ability to work well with others; the ability to blossom without being in the limelight as the "top dog"; the balance and commitment to pursue personal and practice goals without detriment to either; and the desire to be a team player for the pursuit and accomplishment of the greater practice purpose.

Sound ideal? Certainly. But the possibility of building such a team is high when the time and care is invested in the interview process. Remember, there are numerous hidden costs in personnel turnover. The obvious costs are the time wasted and the dollars required to hire and train. But there are other costs as well, such as the morale of employees and patients, image perception factors, and the drain it has on the practice productivity.

Don't rush the process of hiring. Take the time to search, interview, re-interview, compare, test them out, and select. It will pay off in the long run.

Where to Find Good Employees

There are many sources to explore in seeking out qualified individuals for your practice. The following is a partial listing. Given some time and thought you can probably think of many more, based on your particular lifestyle, circle of friends, associates, etc.

- Patients (may be a candidate or know of someone who could be)
- Staff (recommendations by team members often make great candidates since they know the practice, the values and norms, and the kind of person who would work well with the team)
- Dental supply representatives and other suppliers
- Other dentists (ask your colleagues if they know of anyone considering a change, or if they have recently interviewed qualified people they didn't hire)
- Friends and acquaintances (your social circle)
- Newspaper classified advertisement (help wanted) Note: You will get your best return by including a phone number in the ad. If there are many applicants in the market you may want to consider a post office box reply. This, however, discourages those people who are concerned it might be a blind ad for their current employer. Thus, your chances of attracting those people who are unemployed or untrained will increase, and those who are currently employed will decrease.
- Bulletin type announcements in various newsletters or bulletins (church, dental society, etc.)
- Employment agencies, including temporary help agencies

There are many sources of applicants beyond the obvious. Think about your lifestyle and your community and determine for yourself the various sources you can draw on for potential employees.

Chapter 9

PLANNING THE INTERVIEW

The planning process is key to laying the foundation for successful hiring decisions and is a valuable investment. This must happen long before the applicant arrives for the interview. The following process will help you formulate your planning process.

Identify the job requirements and performance standards. Write them down in an *accurate job description* if you don't already have one. Focus on the major responsibilities and the skill, education and experience requirements for each position. This is important in being able to develop meaningful, specific, job-related questions for the interview.

If you have yet to develop a job description for each position, get your team involved and helping in the process. Have them actually begin their own job description. They may need to carry a pad and pencil around for a week to monitor and write down their daily and weekly activities. Have them also identify activities that are done on a monthly basis as well. Job descriptions help eliminate stress on employees that results from role overload, role conflict, and role ambiguity. Don't hire someone and try to fit her into your needs...the shoe just may not fit and it will be uncomfortable. Know what you need, then interview until you find it.

The basics of a job description should include:

- Areas of responsibility (this includes tasks such as scheduling appointments, posting charges and payments, confirming patients, seating patients, sterilizing instruments, room set-ups and take-downs, etc.)
- Goals (effective booking, correctly posted charges, eliminating no shows and late cancellations, etc.)
- Priority of duties

Performance standards should also be included when considering the job description. Performance standards are the ongoing performance criteria that must be met continually in the course of the work. They tell *how* the work will be measured. Standards are usually expressed quantitatively and refer to such things as:

- attendance
- weekly production level
- collections percentages
- percentage of pre-appointed hygiene appointments
- number of prophy's scheduled
- safety standards
- how soon the phone should be answered (how many rings)
- production rates

Another part of performance standards is the manner in which you expect the work to be done or behavioral expectations. These are usually subjective factors such as a caring manner, giving a patient full attention and making them feel like the most important patient in the practice, listening, and working as a team. Consider including in your performance standards that a team effort is expected from all employees to help each other and the doctor, to care for the patients, and to help build the image and overall health of the practice. Job descriptions should also be written in such a way that employees understand what they do is *expected to add value* for the patients.

Involving your team members in developing the job descriptions and performance standards encourages them to take responsibility and become involved in the decision making process.

Identify applicant requirements. In other words, know who you want to hire. Before you can begin the process of seeking out new employees, it is important that you first have a profile of the individual you are looking for. Without the profile, you might not recognize the perfect individual even if he or she is staring you in the face! When you have a position to fill, it is tempting to hire the first person who can breathe, walk, and talk at the same time, especially when you feel pressed for time. But don't do it.

Ask yourself and your team first, "What kind of person will best complement our staff?" Consider such factors as whether the position requires an innovative, creative approach or a more systematic, methodical approach. Also identify any characteristics and skills needed to complement the team or compensate for current areas of weakness. Know what you are looking for. Here are some of the basics:

Attitude. The front office personnel can be of assistance here. Have them engage in conversation with the applicant while the person is waiting for the interview. Obviously this front desk person must be coached on how to elicit information without giving information that will be telegraphed back in the interview.

People skills. Dentistry is about people and building relationships, with trust as the foundation. Although technical skills such as clinical skills or skills in scheduling are important, these can be taught or refined. The people part is much more difficult.

Many in dentistry have been reluctant to hire people without dental experience for non-clinical positions. Yet, many great employees are found in other industries that do wonderful customer service training of their employees. These great customer service people are good prospects for dental front desk positions. It is important to be able to train them and bring them up to "dental awareness" quickly, however. The front desk person needs to be quite knowledgeable in order to handle the phone and inquiries effectively. She is truly your ambassador for the practice.

Financial coordinators require people with communication skills to discuss money issues. Often the reasons people don't pay their bills is because there has been a problem in communication. People trained in other industries to handle financial matters can be a tremendous asset in your practice with their ability to approach and sell patients on the subject of dental services and fees. Because of their previous business experience handling financial matters, they have a matter of fact philosophy in discussing financial matters, and understand the necessity of paying for services rendered.

Consider hiring individuals with a strong desire to move into the dental field who already have developed people skills, who communicate caring and compassion, and who have a desire to serve. You can teach them the technical parts of the position. Obviously, where education is required, the individual must have completed the requirements.

Ability to remain balanced under pressure. Certainly there are stresses in every practice, every day: to stay on schedule, handle emergencies, deal with difficult patients, complete difficult procedures, etc. The team works together more smoothly and the day progresses much more easily when the team members are capable of dealing with the normal pressures of dentistry gracefully.

Lifelong learner. When each member of your team is a willing learner, moving the practice forward is an exciting process. As long as each person knows, understands, and accepts that dentistry is changing, and will continue to change, you will be in a much better position to do what is necessary to move with those changes to maintain your position in the market, to maintain the practice of your dreams, etc.

Team player. An individual who is not a team player will cause heartache for the practice. Every member of the team must be willing to work together. Patients will "feel" the individual who is not part of the team and the practice image will be negatively affected. Just as important, the individual who works "outside the team" makes the entire workload heavier for the rest of the team. There is no place in a well-run dental practice for the "hold-out", regardless of the position or how skilled the individual.

Flexibility. The successful and happiest individuals in dentistry today are those who have the capability of adjusting to changes and conditions around them. The tremendous changes we are experiencing in the industry will continue in the years ahead, and team members must be able to respond accordingly.

Appearance. This includes neatness. Your patients will judge you by what they see in your employees. People who project the image you want are very valuable to your practice.

Personality. It is important that you hire someone with whom you can work, and who will work well with the rest of the team. Employees must be able to interact well with the variety of patients you have in your practice.

Experience. You must determine whether you want only an experienced employee, or if you are willing to take someone with the right attitude and people skills and invest the time and money to train. It can be advantageous to hire those without dental experience who have a burning desire to move into the field of dentistry.

The myth of the job of a good manager or leader is to motivate. In actuality, we cannot motivate anyone...all we can do is provide an environment conducive to lighting the spark that must already exist within the individual. Motivation means *to be led from within by values, beliefs, feelings, and emotions.* Each person is motivated by their own values, beliefs, feelings, and emotions.

Find the individual who has a commitment to the same values and philosophy you have. When you do, the motivation will follow closely within the proper environment. By asking appropriate questions, determine whether or not the individual could support your vision and mission. Don't tell her first what your vision and mission is and ask if she feels or believes that way. That's telegraphing. Ask her questions first. (See Appendix for questions.)

As a child in the third grade my parents allowed me to take accordion lessons and I loved it. I loved being able to take my accordion with me wherever I went so I could play. But when I was in the sixth grade my mother, who had always wanted to play the piano, decided it would be great if I could play the piano. My accordion lessons were stopped and piano lessons began. My heart wasn't in it...and needless to say, I didn't practice. I wanted to go back to the accordion (which I subsequently did).

That's the way it is in hiring staff. If you hire someone you think has the skills, but doesn't have the desire, you will be fighting a losing battle all the way. When you find someone who is truly committed, it is a great match and becomes a wonderful experience.

Identify each of the factors important to you in the individual you hire. Know what you need and want *before* the interviews begin. If you haven't gone through this process before, don't do it alone. Get your other team members involved. Ask them to help you identify what the team needs and wants. Get their input. When you do, they will more easily accept the outcome.

Rather than leave the process of identifying the profile to chance, I utilize a performance tool to help me make that assessment in the practices with which I work. The Prep II Job Analysis allows the doctor or other appropriate person to answer a series of questions about a particular position in their practice to identify the profile(s) of the person who would be best suited for the position. It is used to improve human resource management by creating an environment where people are matched to the position for optimal personal effectiveness. With this knowledge, coupled with the Prep I (the questionnaire given to the final applicants to determine their profile) we can provide practices with personality and behavioral stress assessment for potential and current employees to determine the "matchability" factor. This takes a lot of guesswork out of the hiring process.

The importance of finding the right person for each position justifies the time necessary for careful consideration and study. This means taking a close look at your entire profile and assessing, as closely as you can, the match between your profile and the individual applicant.

↗ Appendix A

Develop interview questions. It is important to determine ahead of time the questions you want to ask when interviewing potential employees. Don't go into the interview "winging" it, or you run the risk of asking questions that are illegal and leaving out questions you really want to ask. Although it takes time up front to prepare for the interview, it will save you much frustration and wasted time.

Identify the questions you want to ask. Make sure you do not inquire about marital or family status, nationality, religion, health background, age, or whether or not they have been a recipient of worker's compensation in the past. Note, however, that by being creative you can ask questions that are legal, and at the same time allow you to ascertain many facts about a prospective employee.

Consider both skill and personality requirements. A good job description will be invaluable here. Questions to address the major technical areas as well as interpersonal skills and motivation are important. Ask questions that give you an example of past performance in these areas and how they handled the situation.

Responses to real life situations give useful data that is also somewhat "predictive" of future behavior. Refer to the list of interview questions provided for you in Appendix A. You can develop others appropriate for your practice.

Also consider role-playing a variety of situations with the applicant to see how they respond, or ask situational type questions such as..."What would you do if....." and then give a particular situation. Don't get hung up on the actual words used. Instead, listen for attitude and philosophy. You can train them on the words later if they have the basic philosophy.

Review applications and resumes. This should be done *before* the interview to allow time to digest the information and identify areas you will need to address, and about which you can ask specific questions. Reviewing both these information sources *in advance* will result in a more thorough interview. It will also increase your confidence in your interviewing ability. Whether you review it a day or two in advance, or literally in the time just before you meet with the applicant, make sure you invest the time necessary to do a thorough review of the application and resume and make note of any questions or concerns you want to discuss.

Be sure to notice any gaps in work history or time unaccounted for and ask the applicant about them during the interview. Make sure all previous employment positions are listed. Sometimes applicants will not list positions that were of short duration, or practices where they burned bridges or left negative relationships and conflict behind.

Plan hosting arrangements. Remember, you are both the *buyer* and the *seller* when you are interviewing applicants for your position. If the applicant doesn't have a good feeling initially, you may lose out on having them *consider you* for their career.

Someone should be available to greet applicants when they arrive and make them as comfortable as possible. The interview location should be private and there should be no interruptions. Each individual applicant should be given *undivided attention* during the interview.

Chapter 10

CONDUCTING THE FIRST INTERVIEW

Once the planning process is completed, it is time to conduct the interview. The interview is a focused, directed conversation between two or more people to identify complementary needs and skills. You need an employee...the applicant needs a job. With this focus, the tone should be one of interest and mutual respect.

Actually, the selection process is a courtship period to determine if the marriage will work, and an elimination process for those who do not have what you want and need. During the entire process you will learn about the applicant, his or her qualifications, success potential, strengths and weaknesses, and even pertinent personal factors that come up during the interviews. You will also be informing the applicant about what you have to offer.

1. Establish Rapport. Greet the applicant warmly, offer a firm handshake, provide a cup of coffee or soft drink, and briefly encourage small talk. This will help reduce any anxieties the applicant may be experiencing and help create the atmosphere for a more open, honest and candid discussion. Establishing rapport is very important and until you do you will most likely not get to know who the applicant really is. Use whatever you know about the person....current job, school, hobby, or anything else... to break the ice. Perhaps she was referred by someone you know. Ask how she knows that person. By your body language, facial gestures, tone of voice, and your focused attention, let her know you are interested, not judgmental. When people feel they are being judged they tend to tense up and close the door to *open* communication.

As part of the rapport building, find out the applicant's time constraints. Does she have time to complete a good, solid interview with you, or is she running to another appointment. Both of you need to be able to give your full focus to the interview.

2.   *Present a brief, broad overview of the position.* The tendency for most interviewers is to *telegraph* by talking too much and communicating exactly what type of individual is needed for the job. Telegraphing tells the applicant what you want *before* you find out whether or not she has it. The tendency, when this happens, is for the applicant to repeat back to you exactly what you said, thus giving you an inaccurate picture of herself. This happens most frequently when the interview has not been planned, and the interviewer is at a loss in knowing where to go next. At this stage of the interview, present *only an overview* of the practice, patient base, and the position.

Your prepared questions should be used as a guide, not a rigid structure. When the applicant's response raises additional questions or curiosity, feel free to probe more deeply by asking clarifying questions. Having situational questions as part of the written application form, requiring the applicant to think and then put the responses in writing, eliminates time in the interview. There is value, however, in asking a few situational or behavioral questions during the interview to allow you to see how the person might respond under pressure.

When asking these questions, be sure you allow silence as part of the process. Sometimes, especially with behavioral questions, the applicant will need time to think of specific examples. Allow that time without feeling the need to keep a constant flow of conversation. If you are comfortable with silence, the applicant will also feel more comfortable. Perhaps a lead-in to the "okayness" of silent time for thinking might be, "I know these are tough questions, but I ask them of all applicants. Just take your time." Then rest quietly, sit back and let the applicant think.

3.   *Observe non-verbal cues and behavior...both yours and the applicant's.* Your non-verbal behavior can influence the outcome and progression of the interview. Squenched eyebrows, obvious tensing, and other physical signs of your disapproval may cause the applicant to steer clear of the area and give a response she feels is more in line with what she *thinks* you want to hear. That's part of the telegraphing! A slight nod, rather than signs of disapproval or judgment, encourages the applicant to continue the discussion of the topic in question.

The applicant's non-verbal behavior is also important. For example, if she seems uncomfortable in discussing her relationship with the last supervisor or doctor, probe more deeply. *"You seem a little uneasy talking about your supervisor. How would you describe your relationship with him/her?"* As you do, make sure you remain neutral in your tone and delivery. Then stay present to and focused on the applicant. Important clues can be missed otherwise. Be attuned to the value placed on what she talks about and watch for emerging attitudes about her job, her previous or current employer, the dental field as a whole, her self-esteem, and confidence level.

During the search for our hygienist, one temporary seemed to do quite well in the two days she was in the practice. The existing staff members felt good about her and the patients seemed to like her. We already knew that she, too, was searching for a full time position. At the end of her first couple days, she was approached about her interest in applying for the position. When she said she was interested, she was given our normal application (consisting of a general application, followed by several case situations asking how she would handle or respond to those situations).

After looking at the application she handed it to Norm and said, "I won't   fill this out. This is demeaning. You already know how I work and that should be enough." She wouldn't even complete the routine application section! That raised questions about this person. Could we count on her to be flexible? Would she really perform as a part of the team, or would she live in her own world? Would she accept suggestions or ideas from any other team member, including the doctor?

Remember, we can think faster than we speak, making distractions easy. But it is important to listen completely and remain aware. Give the applicant your undivided attention. Listen actively to the questions asked, the answers given, and the non-verbal behavior. Lean forward slightly, maintain appropriate eye contact (but don't stare and cause uneasiness). Provide feedback to continue the interview or responses to questions by saying, *"I see,"* or *"Tell me more"* or *"How did you feel about that?"*

All feedback responses should be verbalized *without implying that you either agree or disagree*. Ask clarifying questions, and avoid fidgeting behavior or constant clock watching.

4. *Take brief notes.* This allows you to summarize and make note of key points for later consideration and evaluation. Once the applicant is gone, and especially after you have interviewed several, it becomes difficult to remember what it was you liked or disliked, or to identify the red and green flags. Don't take voluminous notes or the applicant may become uncomfortable. Simply get down the most significant points you want to remember.

5. *Allow the applicant to ask questions.* By encouraging questions you reinforce an open, honest response. The match you are trying to achieve is on both sides; it must be good for both you and the applicant. Therefore, the applicant needs to be allowed time and consideration for her questions.

6. *Summarize.* Review briefly and summarize what you heard the applicant saying about her interests, abilities, skills and even concerns. This will help ensure the picture you have of the applicant is accurate. This gives the applicant and yourself the opportunity to confirm or eliminate assumptions and clarify perceptions.

7. *Sell the job realistically.* During the final stages of initial interviewing, the career opportunity can be described in greater detail. *After* you feel you have a pretty good understanding of the applicant, get into the specifics of the job and all her questions.

That way you won't be telegraphing responses that will be repeated back to you.

It is important not to make promises you can't keep or oversell the positive aspects of the position without giving due consideration to any drawbacks. Help the applicant think about how the position fits into her overall career objectives. If it is not a good match, it is good to identify and discuss it now...not two or three months after she has been hired.

**8. *Conclude by letting the applicant know what will happen next.* Let the applicant know your interview process. Will there be other interviews? Will you have other team members interview final applicants? When is a hiring decision expected to be made? It is also important to find out whether or not the applicant has other offers pending. This is especially important if you feel she is a well-qualified candidate for your position.

Thank the applicant for her time. Be sure to clearly communicate who makes the next move. If you are not really sure whether or not she is a likely candidate, you might ask her to consider all you discussed and get back to you by a specific date to let you know of her interest in the position. If you feel this is one of your finalists, schedule a second interview or let her know when she will be contacted for another interview. Another option is to tell her you are very interested in her and you would like her to take some time to consider the position and contact you if she would like to pursue it. Be sure to communicate clearly that you are looking for the right match, from the perspective of all individuals involved, and that's why it is important for her to give careful consideration to what has been discussed.

If you are think you are not interested in this person, thank her for her time, tell her you have several interviews yet to complete, and that she will be contacted in the event she is considered for a second interview.

Remember, in the initial interview you are only trying to get a general impression in order to determine if you want to see that person again. *Right now you are looking for weaknesses and reasons not to hire*...as well as strengths and reasons to hire. Obvious and significant weaknesses that are inappropriate for the position will help you eliminate the applicant early in the process so you can invest valuable interview time with more promising candidates.

More than one interview should be accomplished before any hiring decision is made. People returning for second and third interviews often begin to let you see more of the "real" them. It has been said that the closest a person ever comes to perfection is on a resume. You want to get beyond that...and it will take time with the applicant to do so.

Chapter 11

EVALUATING THE APPLICANT

Immediately after the applicant has left the interview record additional observations. Identify and note in writing the specific behavioral traits and qualities that will influence your hiring decision. The objective is to determine the applicant's success potential *in your practice.* Remember, it is *your* practice you are concerned about and how the individual would be as a member of *your* team....not someone else's. A person who would be great in your best friend's practice on the other side of town may not be the best individual for your team and your practice.

Now is the time to compare all the requirements of the job and the applicant's capabilities. This is best done right after the interview *before going on to another applicant or other tasks,* while your memory is still fresh. Waiting causes fading of memory! If the applicant meets or exceeds the requirement, make that notation. When you have completed all your first interviews, determine which applicants you want to see for a second interview. Compare each person to the qualifications of the other qualified applicants to determine who seems to be the best match for your practice.

Realize that over-hiring can be just as big a mistake as under-hiring. An overly qualified person may be bored or feel limited by the position, while an under-qualified applicant might feel stressed and unable to meet the job requirements.

Check References

Before you conduct the final interview, make your decision, or offer the position to an applicant, a complete check of the applicant's background and job experience through a series of meaningful reference inquiries is vitally important. Often this key responsibility, if not omitted completely, is treated most casually. This lack of thoroughness can easily result in poor hiring decisions. Be aware, however, that you must ask and receive permission from the applicant before you check references. If you receive any negative information, be sure to keep this confidential. Otherwise, the person you spoke with can be held liable for defamation of character. If the applicant asks you, tell her it is your policy not to divulge any information, positive or negative, received in checking references.

If possible, talk with the applicant's previous employer. Describe the position available and try to get any input you can as to how the applicant will "fit." By briefly describing the position, the person may be more willing to be honest and provide you with good feedback. If you have specific concerns about the applicant, mention them and ask for any input the previous employer may be able to give. This approach often elicits more information than simply saying, "I am calling about Cathy Sharp. What kind of recommendation can you give?" And always ask, at the end, *"Would you rehire this person?"* A "no" to this may be a major red flag. See Appendix B for suggested questions in reference checking.

Keep in mind this important guideline throughout the entire process: ***Never allow yourself to jump to conclusions or make a decision until all the facts are in.*** This is easier said than done, because when we like a person we almost instinctively and immediately decide we want this person. It's love at first sight, without allowing the courtship period to get to know the person before a decision is made. This is called the *halo effect.* Coupled with the urgency to hire a new person, it may cause you to magnify strengths and overlook weaknesses. When this happens you may be in for a rude awakening and an early dissolution of the relationship if the person is hired.

Check the Current Employer

One of the most difficult references to obtain, yet one of the most important, is the company with whom the applicant is currently employed. There are three ways to check this source:

• Ask the applicant if it would be possible to speak with either the doctor, supervisor (if different) or another person in the practice who couldappropriately comment on her performance, and not jeopardize her position with the practice.

• Ask the applicant to suggest someone with whom she worked in the current practice, but who is no longer with the company.

• Make your job offer conditional. That is, make it a condition of the job offer that the applicant will receive a satisfactory reference from her current employer, and check with that employer after the applicant has given her resignation.

There is considerable risk in hiring someone who will not accept one of these proposals and there is nothing that can replace a thorough reference check. Although it is not foolproof, not doing it creates an unnecessary risk. Doing so will prevent disappointment, frustration and needless effort, time and money spent in hiring people who are not appropriate for the position in your practice.

During the interview process for our administrative assistant some time ago we interviewed a person who obviously was well-qualified from an experience standpoint. She had worked in a well-known, well-respected practice for fourteen years. In the interview, however, it was discovered that she was fired by one of the doctors in the practice. For other reasons, we decided not to consider her for a second interview and as a result, did not do any reference checking. Some time later, however, Norm was speaking with her previous employer and found out that this person had embezzled at least $16,000 from the practice!

This is a perfect example of why reference checks are important. Talking with this applicant, she appeared competent, confident, and willing to do the job. She presented herself very well, was very articulate, and very attractive. We didn't, however, feel that her personality was appropriate for our practice and did not continue further into the interview process. It would have been easy to overlook reference checks with this individual if her personality had been more acceptable to our team. If that had been the case, we could have made a very big hiring mistake.

Chapter 12

Subsequent Interviews

We've already indicated the importance of having more than one interview before an applicant is hired. Second and subsequent interviews may be built around any number of factors:

- Obtain additional information you failed to get or didn't have time to get in the first interview.
- Have each of your staff members spend a few minutes with the applicant. Have them identify questions before they go into the interview so they can make this productive time. Then get input from your team about their feelings, hesitations, concerns, positive comments, etc. This is very effective and helps the team work together as a team...and feel a part of the decision making in something that impacts them tremendously.
- Answer any questions the applicant may have.
- Provide a more in-depth explanation of what your expectations are (after getting information from the applicant first, to minimize telegraphing).
- Utilize any personality profiles or other appropriate and legal testing tools.

Again, profiles or instruments for testing can be a tremendous aid in interviewing and selection. Earlier I mentioned the job analysis profile, Prep II, that I normally use with my clients. Additionally I use the Prep I Profile to determine whether or not the applicant fits the profile that would best work with a particular team in a particular practice. This profile allows us to better understand the behavioral tendencies of an individual. From it we can learn many things about the applicant that will help us in our decision: the natural style of behavior, behavioral changes a person is currently making, what morale is indicated by the behavioral change, what the long-term and short-term stress levels are, the total coping energy available, the individual's predictable first impression personality, and the problem-solving and communication styles of this person.

However you choose to structure your interviews, understand the importance of seeing the applicant more than one time...in fact more than two times is preferable.

Working Interviews

Chairside assistant and hygienist positions lend themselves well to a working interview. Have the applicant work for you for a full day to see how well she relates to the rest of the team, how comfortable you feel with her, what her actual skill level is, and how she deals with pressure (there's sure to be some the first day!). Be sure you don't expect her to work for nothing. Make the investment and pay a fair wage. Remember, you are establishing right up front the kind of person you are. If you've been telling the applicant all along that you are generous and everyone works together, and then you ask that person to work for nothing, you have just created a question concerning the principle of integrity in the applicant's mind...of congruency between what you say you are and do, and what you actually are and do.

The Final or "Selection" Interview

The final interview, the selection interview, whether it is the second or fifth, has three main objectives:

- To give you a final look at the applicant as you examine her background, attitudes and qualifications in depth.
- To give the applicant a final look as you answer her questions and provide further information about the position and your practice.
- To offer her the position if you like what you see, hear, and have discovered.

Sometimes you may be unpleasantly surprised when you see an applicant again, even though you were favorably impressed in an earlier interview. This discrepancy may be due to a number of factors. Perhaps the applicant was unconsciously compared with a few obviously unqualified applicants which made her look good. It may be because you have unconsciously lowered your standards, feeling pressed to hire someone immediately. It may be because the applicant relaxed her concern over her appearance or behavior, thinking you were already "sold" because you brought her back.

Whatever the reason, one thing is very clear. It is difficult, if not impossible, to make a purely objective appraisal of a person. Actually this is good. If you dislike a person it will be very difficult for you to work with, train, direct, motivate, coach, advise, listen to, and trust her. This is vitally important, especially in dentistry, because many practices are small enough that every person is working closely with every other person every day.

During this final interview, a good opener is *"What was it that prompted you to return for this interview?"* Actually, this is a great question for any second and subsequent interview. This will give you some indication of the thoughts, feeling level, what she likes about your practice and opportunity, and whether or not she simply hasn't had any other successful job interviews or offers. All these will give you further information for your decision.

Between the last interview and this one, the applicant will no doubt have discussed the opportunity with her spouse, parents, friends, and other people in dentistry. As a result, she may have additional questions. Allow time for these.

The selection interview is very important. It is important that you review the information you have about the applicant, your earlier notes and observations, and the job requirements. Since the selection interview should never be the first interview, you will have taken the time to check references and may have additional questions based on any red or green lights that were flagged based on information you uncovered.

After all the questions are answered on both sides (yours and hers), if you still feel confident this is the person you want to hire, again clarify the position. Make sure there is a clear understanding of what it involves and what you expect. Discuss other factors such as dress codes and uniform requirements, employee benefits, training, how she will be paid, and any other expectations. Before offering the job, make sure the applicant understands the limitations and the promotion potential (if that is a concern) and feels comfortable about both. When this is clear the risk of over-hiring or under-hiring can be reduced. This thorough clarification of all factors is vitally important to ensure that questions don't arise later causing the applicant to feel she wasn't given full disclosure of the position. Full disclosure of all aspects, including expectations, establishes a clear track to run on. It will make working with your new employee much easier and sets the stage for a great relationship and effective performance reviews along the way.

Finally, when you have made your decision and the applicant has accepted, give her a copy of your employee manual, welcome her aboard, and clarify the starting date and any other necessary information. Then plan for her orientation to get her off to a successful start.

Common Errors in Employee Selection

Several common errors can undermine the interview process. Listed below are some of the more frequent errors and how to eliminate them.

Inadequate screening

• Determine the specification for the position before you advertise and recruit. Make sure this is done *before* you look at applications so you will not be fooled by impressive, but ill-suited, resumes and applicants.

• Establish a checklist, then go through each resume and disqualify those not meeting specifications.

• Don't be swayed or taken in by the "halo" effect of applicants who write persuasively, who call or visit to ask more about the position, who magnify their practical experience, or who ignore your requests for experience but try to convince you their education is enough.

Inadequate preparation

If, during the initial interview, you immediately ask questions that are already answered in the resume or application, you are not prepared. After the interview is over you will know no more about the applicant than when you read the application. Before the interview:

• Determine the job requirements
• Examine the resume and application thoroughly
• Plan and organize pertinent interview questions
• Arrange for a private place to conduct the interview

Failure to probe for greater understanding

Interviewers with little experience, or those who do not feel comfortable interviewing, often accept inadequate responses to questions. They will accept superficial or ambiguous answers, fail to ask for clarification, and then make incorrect assumptions. Lead-ins for probing include statements like:

• Could you explain what you meant by...?
• Please tell me more about...?
• How did you feel about that?

Unintentional "leading" or telegraphing of "desired" answers

By leading the applicant to a particular response you will not know whether you are obtaining accurate information or getting responses that you have influenced by your tone of voice, what you have said, or by your non-verbal clues. One major mistake is telling the applicant about the job and the job requirements *before* you do the interviewing.

Let the applicant answer in her own words. Even if she is groping for a word, let her do her own talking instead of "helpfully" completing her sentences with *your* words.

Give the applicant time to think about your questions instead of adding "in other words" interpretations of your own. Here are some examples of leading and telegraphing that should *not* be used:

You do enjoy working with people, don't you?
You wouldn't mind working late some evenings, would you?
I'd say that's a good reason for leaving a job.
I know what you mean. I feel that way too.

Dominating the interview

Dominating the interview usually results from one of three things: not being prepared, nervousness, or not knowing when to stop talking.

You learn very little about the applicant if you do all the talking. Your job is to create an atmosphere that will encourage the applicant to talk. Learn to lead the discussion, not dominate it. A good rule of thumb is to conduct the interview so the applicant does 70% of the talking.

Failing to listen

Actively listen. Keep good eye contact and observe the applicant for clues and signals, and get feedback if you have missed a point or do not understand. Listen without interrupting, preaching, lecturing, or judging. Listen to what is being said rather than thinking about your next question.

Preaching, lecturing, judging

Certain comments can suggest an unfavorable attitude on your part to a remark made by the applicant. Comments like these can embarrass the applicant and create obstacles for obtaining further information. They could also result in defensiveness or other emotional reactions that would minimize the effectiveness of the interview. Examples of this type of "commenting" are:

That wasn't the best thing to do, was it?
You've learned how to handle that situation now, haven't you?
That really wasn't the best reason for quitting, was it?
You don't really feel that way, do you?

Failing to ask good questions

When you ask questions, keep these general guidelines in mind:

• Ask one question at a time. Two or three-part questions should be avoided.
• Ask neutral questions (don't telegraph your feelings or what you want to hear).
• Rephrase questions if the answer is not clear or you're not sure you understand.
• Ask, "How, what, why and tell me" questions for probing, not "Don't you think" type questions.
• Don't ask questions that can be answered yes or no. These are dead-end questions and don't allow you to obtain much useful information. Yes/No questions should be used only when you want a narrow, limited response and are looking specifically for a Yes/No only answer.
• Always have a clear purpose behind your questions. Don't be redundant, repeat questions, or ask irrelevant questions just to keep the interview going because you can't think of anything else to say at the time.

Taking voluminous notes...or no notes at all

Make brief, pertinent notes during the interview. Make more detailed notes immediately following. Memory fades and a few notes are important for later recall.

Poor attitude on the interviewer's part

Be sure you don't come across as abrasive, condescending, argumentative, indifferent, or irritated. Watch your tone of voice.

Never put the applicant down. This creates bad feelings toward you and your practice in general, and will cause your applicant to "clam up" and not give you the information you need to make an accurate, fair appraisal.

Don't prejudge or be unduly biased by an applicant before you gather information. If the applicant initially impressed you strongly, either positively or negatively, do not assume all other factors are in line with this first impression.

Premature evaluation and selection

It is difficult to maintain an objective attitude throughout the process of interviewing all the applicants, but by doing so, you will be more likely to make the best choice. First impressions can be inaccurate and assumptions incorrect. When you rely only on hunches, or allow yourself to make premature decisions, you risk the possibility of creating a self-fulfilling prophecy. Also, if you interview two or three applicants in a row who do not have the appropriate skills, experience level, or other qualifications, it becomes easy to look at the "best of the worst' and end up making a faulty hiring decision.

Keep your attitude open during the time you do *all* the interviews, and then check against the job requirements for a "match." Don't fall victim to hiring "the best of the worst." *Reacting puts us in the crisis mode; proactivity keeps us in the choice mode.* Relax. Use temporary help until you find the right person, and commit yourself to search until you truly believe you have found the right person.

Chapter 13

Effectively Integrating the New Employee

Strategic hiring is critical to developing a healthy team for the practice. Once a new team member is hired, however, a well-structured orientation is extremely important to minimize turnover. An employee is never more focused, open and teachable than on the first day of a new job. They want to do well. They are open to learn.

Unfortunately, in many practices the orientation is nothing more than saying hello in the morning huddle and showing them where their "tools" are, and expecting them to go at it! That's not an orientation. The new employee orientation should include the following.

Welcome the new employee. The doctor or office manager is responsible for introducing the new employee to the entire team...every single member. The introduction should include clear communication of how fortunate you believe you are to have this person on the team. Tell of this person's background or whatever you feel makes this person the right choice for the position. Build up the new employee. Unless you and your office manager, if you have one, stimulate acceptance by other team members of the new person's credibility, respect, etc., it may or may not happen. When you let your team members know you value this individual and the contribution she can make, you pave the way for that person's acceptance and integration into the team.

It should be noted, however, that if you do not feel this way about your existing employees, they may actually resent your feelings about the new person. If this is the situation in your practice (and deep down you know) then you've got some work to do. You can't expect people to go the extra mile, work as a team, and do whatever it takes to reach practice goals if they don't feel appreciated and believed in by you.

Review, once again, the job description. Make sure you are communicating on the same level.

Review the employee manual. The new employee should have read it by this time. Ask if there are any questions or if anything is unclear. Perhaps have her sign a short statement in her development folder indicating she has read it and will agree to follow it.

Review benefits. Make sure there has been no miscommunication. This includes pay, bonuses, insurance, profit sharing, sick leave/wellness benefit, etc.

Provide an introduction to the physical layout of the office. Show the new employee where everything is located: instruments, dental supplies, office supplies, etc. Where are street clothes and uniforms are kept? If she brings a lunch, where does she put it? Where does she go for a quick break? Where are the morning huddles held? Where are the restrooms...both for patients and staff?

Give your new team member a clear overview of your practice. Review again your philosophy including vision, mission and goals.

Describe your team philosophy. Discuss the values of your practice and how you go about doing what you do. Let her know up front how you work together as a team...what is acceptable behavior, and what is not. Include a discussion on continual improvement and continuing education.

Miscellaneous. Include any other factors or areas you feel are important about your practice, such as safety issues and how you implement the OSHA guidelines.

The purpose of the orientation is to fully integrate the new person into the practice. You want her to feel a part of the team as quickly as possible, and that requires a complete orientation. It's not fair to hire a person and ask her to function at her capacity, to work as an integral member of the team, when she has not been fully introduced.

While this may seem like a lot of work, it will reap you dividends you never anticipated. Don't feel you have to do the entire process yourself, nor complete it in one day. In fact, the more employees you involve in the process the better. Develop a systematic orientation for new employees. Write it out. Determine who will be responsible for what portion and when. Perhaps you'll want to break these eight areas into one or two weeks, covering one or more areas a day. In your plan, determine who will be responsible for covering each topic and on what day. Then make sure the people you have doing each section of the orientation is well-prepared to do a thorough job.

We all know how important the first impression and the entire new patient process is in getting off to the right start with a new patient. The employee orientation is the equivalent process in hiring new employees.

Where some people manage or try to lead by fear, and find poor results in the long run, the leader who leads out of love will reap bountiful rewards. People who are afraid don't dare perform to the limit of their capabilities. They can't take risks when they are afraid or threatened. They won't go the extra mile when they don't feel truly a part of the team, or feel their position in the practice matters. On the other hand, when there is an atmosphere of loving concern, where people are respected and trusted, they will risk and go the extra mile. As a result they will grow, become more productive, and their potential will blossom. The orientation is a vital part of establishing this atmosphere from the start.

Chapter 14

TRAINING

Once on board, helping all employees grow, and rewarding and recognizing their accomplishments are big factors affecting the individual's success and the overall practice success. One aspect of this is training. Although the interview and orientation process may be exemplary, without ongoing training your team may suffer.

We are already seeing a shortage of qualified dental personnel in all positions. To succeed in dentistry in the 21st century, and to ensure we have top-of-the-line personnel, will require that we *develop* people. If we've not been accustomed to doing this in the past, this will be a major change. Success will come only with the ability to be flexible and change to meet changing conditions. The world is different today, and we must respond to it differently to maintain our current level or achieve new levels of success.

It is incredible how many people, in their personal or professional lives, don't like the results, yet repeat the same things over and over hoping to get different results. Einstein called this insanity! If we don't like our results, we must change the equation. If we have been working with the numbers 2 + 2 and don't like the answer four, then we must change the equation in order to get any other answer. We are very much like that. We can't just move the pieces around in a different order...we must do something differently. And training may be one piece of the equation that will yield much greater results for your practice.

Without proper training you may find it difficult to introduce a new product or service. Team members often openly resist the new product, new equipment, ideas for service, etc. without training. On the other hand, when team members are properly trained, they will better accept the new introduction. As a result they will inform, educate, and motivate patients so there is greater patient acceptance where appropriate.

Training empowers employees. Often we expect our employees to know what to do, and exactly how we want it to be done, but never give them the tools or show them what we expect. This results in frustration, anxiety and distress that drains energy and eventually leads to burnout. It neutralizes the power that *could* turn your practice into the practice of your dreams.

Many doctors have been reluctant to train their people because they are afraid of losing their employees to another practice. Some feel they can't spend the money and others feel it takes too much time. The reality is that dental practices with ongoing training actually have happier employees and they tend to attract and keep better employees than practices without training.

Training builds the self-esteem of team members. It also builds morale and attitude, helps reduce turnover, and builds the team by increasing understanding and communication. Training can also reduce potential liability by preventing accidents because of greater awareness.

Often in the past we have tended to think of technical training when we spoke of training, and felt that was all that is needed. Not so. Some of the greatest morale boosters and confidence builders have to do with personal growth training that occurs. Identifying an employee's strengths and building them even stronger is important. Building *beyond* them is just as important.

It is short sighted to believe that all the information needed to make your practice function effectively today, as well as to continue its' journey solidly on target into the future, exists in the current collective knowledge and experience of the team members. Be open to new ideas. Allow yourself to think beyond the self-imposed, imaginary boundaries of the past. Attend continuing education courses for broader understanding as often as possible, and include your team. For example, if you are attending an esthetic dentistry seminar you might think the only people who would profit from it would be you and your assistant. Not so. What about the incredible selling position your front desk person has, as well as the hygienist? When they understand more about esthetic dentistry they can get excited about it. And when they get excited about it, they will help sell your patients on the benefits.

Think about including your team more often in seminars you attend. Bring speakers and practice management consultants into your practice to conduct training sessions, put energy into meetings, or to even conduct a mid-week or week-end retreat for your staff. Look into continuing education courses at local community colleges or universities.

Develop a library for your team members to use for personal and professional development to encourage lifetime learning. We have included many books, audio tapes, and video tapes in our practice library for use by our employees. These cover a wide variety of topics including: how to develop increased skills specific to dentistry or the dental office; personal development (attitude, communication, interpersonal relationships and other related subjects); marriage enrichment and family development (we believe a person who is happy at home has much more to offer the practice and will also be a happier employee); team development; and leadership development.

Abe Lincoln once said, "If I had six hours to chop down a tree, I'd spend the first four hours sharpening the axe." Sharpening the axe, in this case, is training your staff. One of the greatest inefficiencies in a dental practice today is untrained staff. If you wait for a good time to get around to it, it will probably never happen. Schedule it, just like you expect your patients to schedule their treatment. And realize that this should be an ongoing part of your practice. Finally, make sure your training and development evolves from your values, vision, and mission of the practice.

Chapter 15

PERSONAL AND PROFESSIONAL DEVELOPMENT SESSIONS

I am a firm believer that each employee should be given individual attention in what I call the PPDS, or the Personal and Professional Development Session. This is the corollary to the more well known performance review. These sessions can be a tremendous help in moving employees from *what they do* to *what they can do*...tapping into more of their potential. If we feel there is a lack of personal responsibility and initiative with some employees, it may be because our performance review systems have not been designed to *develop* our employees. Employees are much more easily motivated by using the PPDS than by a traditional performance review, which all too often becomes a session focused on '"what is wrong, what I want, and how I expect it changed."

Personal and Professional Development Sessions are development sessions of the whole person. They are two-way dialogues between the doctor (or office manager) and employee about the employee's past, present, and future job performance. The discussions help you both understand what is expected and how the employee's performance compares with those expectations. They help employees identify their strengths, develop their talents, work on their weaknesses, and actually enjoy their work more.

Approximately 25% of the session should be spent on the past and present, where you have been and are right at this moment, and 75% is spent on *where you are going* and *how you are going to get there*. It is important to recognize that the 25% is only to help us figure out where or how we can head in an even better direction. It is not meant to be a "raking over the coals" session. Because that's what many performance review sessions have become, many persons conducting reviews and the employees being reviewed have learned to fear, or at least dislike, review sessions.

Remember this: the review session should never be the first time an employee hears about something she did wrong, a mistake she made, or what you don't like. These kinds of issues should be dealt with *at the time they occur.* When these kinds of problems or complaints are stacked up, waiting for the review, employees will always live in fear of the review, wondering day after day if they have done something they will be "jumped" for later. This creates a very negative and disempowering environment. In this environment an employee holds back suggestions, pulls back from the growth-producing risk activities, and loses enthusiasm, spirit, and creativity. The practice will suffer as a result.

It is a known fact that every person operates below his or her actual potential and as such, human resources are being wasted both for the individual and for the practice. It is the leader's job to stimulate employees to raise the level of their performance and to provide an atmosphere that is conducive to this behavior. The PPDS provides the forum in which this can be identified, monitored and communicated.

Most employees want two questions answered: "How am I doing" and "What can I do to improve." Too often we fail to convey this information. Studies show that a high percentage of employees don't know how they are doing on the job simply because they are not told. This results in exceptional employees not being aware of their strengths, and therefore they may or may not be consistent in what they do or how they do it. Additionally, if they feel their efforts are unappreciated they may lose motivation, become bitter, and even begin searching for another job where they *feel* appreciated. On the other hand, marginal employees are unaware of their shortcomings and may assume that silence means approval. Most assuredly, they will not have the tools to maximize their potential.

To successfully generate positive changes all Personal and Professional Development Sessions must provide four things: (1) agreement by both the employee and supervisor about the direction the employee is headed; (2) what changes are needed to get there; (3) the belief by both people that change is possible; and (4) a mutually agreed upon plan of action to accomplish the change.

Who Should Conduct the Session?

The most effective sessions are conducted by the *immediate supervisor.* In a small dental practice this would usually be the doctor; in a larger practice this might be the office manager. The immediate supervisor is in close working relationship with the employee. Morale is often boosted because the employee can sense the supervisor's interest in her and her work. Both people are (or should be) publicly and personally committed to improving performance and solving mutual problems. Introducing a third person to conduct the PPDS makes communication much more difficult, especially when that person is not involved on a day-to-day basis with the employee.

How Often Should a PPDS Be Conducted?

Routine evaluations are made daily in most practices on an informal basis through "ocular inspection." Obviously, when an employee makes a significant mistake or behaves poorly it should be brought to her attention as soon as possible and not stored up for a future PPDS. Sandbagging causes frustration for the employee, builds fear and resentment, and increases the likelihood that bad habits will become ingrained before corrective behavior is begun.

Consider conducting the PPDS at least every three months for the first year, then possibly moving to a semi-annual review if the employee is progressing well. Any time you see a decline in performance, it is fair to move back into more frequent sessions until such time as you feel less frequent sessions are again appropriate. In any event, a PPDS should be conducted no less than annually.

Preparing for the PPDS

It is important that the employee and the doctor (or supervisor)
are prepared in advance for the PPDS. Remember to:

- Set the date at least one week in advance. The
  employee should know when the PPDS will occur
  and against what standards she will be evaluated.

- Ask the employee to prepare for the session. Depending upon the format you choose, you may want to have
  the employee complete a written evaluation as a guideline for discussion.

- Provide an opportunity for the employee to ask
  questions about the upcoming session.

- Explain that the focus will be on the present and
  future, not on the past. The past only has value
  because it helps determine where attention is needed
  to get to where you want to go.

Some questions you may choose to have the employee reflect on
and write down:

- How am I doing according to my job description and
  performance standards?
- What critical abilities does my job require? To what
  extent do I fulfill them?
- Does my present job make use of my skills and abilities?
- How could I become more productive?
- What have I done since my last PPDS to prepare myself
  for more responsibility?
- What new goals and standards should be established
  for the next PPDS period? Do any need to be modified
  or deleted?

The PPDS should be a session both you and the employee look
forward to. This is not the place to get out a black list of all the

things that have gone wrong since the last session. This is her private time with you, time to identify how she can better fulfill her role in the practice, and how she can also meet her own goals for personal and professional development in the process.

It is important to create an environment that supports and encourages; an environment where each and every individual feels good about their contribution and their accomplishment; an environment where people not only want to go to work, but feel worthwhile and fulfilled by being there. The PPDS, conducted effectively, will help create this kind of environment.

What Should Be Accomplished in the PPDS?

A very basic principle applies to all personal and professional development sessions: Emphasis should be on the present and future, not on the past or what has already happened. What is done is done, and the only benefit of reliving it is what it can teach us for the future.

As we discuss various aspects of the PPDS, keep in mind that there is no magic formula or "one right way." The format that follows, however, is what I have found to be effective in many dental practices, as well as in other businesses. The actual goals of the session should be to:

1. Check how well the employee has met expectations and followed through on the previously agreed upon plan of action (from the prior session).

2. Identify poor work habits and behavior before they become habit. Remember: they should have been brought up at the time you became aware of them. This is a review and there should be no "sandbagged" items for you to bring up. It is appropriate, however, to discuss how the employee is doing on areas identified prior to the PPDS as needing work.

3. Recognize and praise what the employee is doing well.

4. Anticipate any problems or needs before they arise.

5. Determine wants and needs the employee has for continued development.

6. Determine any training or retraining needs.

7. Help the employee plan a course of action for improvement and development.

8. Motivate the employee to put into action what has been identified in the way of opportunities and plans.

Guidelines for Conducting the PPDS

An effective PPDS will result when the above goals are accomplished. The following guidelines will help you to do just that.

Be clear about the purpose. It is impossible to conduct an effective PPDS without a purpose. Make sure the purpose is clear to both you and the employee. People tend to hold back during a session when the purpose is unclear, and defensive behaviors increase (anger, frustration, etc.). The purpose should be to: help the employee become more effective, utilize more of her potential, and continuously develop as a whole person.

Begin by having the employee express her attitudes and outlook. Ask a general question to have her tell you what is on her mind. Discussing this may be the most important part of the session. By doing this first it shows you are interested in her as a person and not just her productivity. Even if the problem can't be solved immediately, at least she has voiced it, allowing her a clearer mind to be more receptive to what follows.

Stay focused. A form for both you and the employee to complete before the PPDS will help you stay on track. Use the form as a tool, but don't let it rule the process.

Before you discuss the person's performance, discuss the job. You may have different ideas about the exact nature of the job than the employee. Review the written job description together and see if it needs revision. Then ask questions such as:

- Do we agree on the job description?
- Which parts of your job do you feel are the most important?
- Do we agree on the prioritization of these?
- Do we agree on the standards by which your work is evaluated?

Ask before you tell. Instead of telling the employee what you think of her work, ask her what she thinks she has done well and what she would like to do better. Most people more readily accept their own criticism than criticism from another. In fact, most will judge themselves more strictly than you will. Review the responses to her written questions and answers.

Do not judge. In fact, the judgment part of the process should be built into the job description and expected performance standards long before any PPDS session takes place. When standards are clear from the beginning the employee knows what she will be measured against, eliminating the need for surprises and you playing "the bad guy." With these clearly identified in advance, the employee becomes her own judge.

A few additional questions may help facilitate this discussion:

- What do you think are your greatest strengths?
- Where do you feel less than competent?
- Do you have any suggestions on how we might help you grow?
- Is there any way that I or someone else could help you do a better job (be more efficient, more effective, more competent)?
- Do I do anything that makes your work harder?
- What do we do in our practice that helps you do your job, that you would like us to continue or perhaps do even more of?
- Is there anything we do that hampers you, minimizes your effectiveness or holds you back?

The last three questions are sometimes difficult for the doctor or supervisor to ask, yet the greatest boost to morale and productivity often comes from these questions.

Be realistic and reflect the way things are. The only way we can get to where we want to go is to know where we are now. This requires honesty on the part of you and the employee. Trust must be the foundation of the relationship before this will happen. Be objective as possible, based on standards rather than opinion, prejudice or bias.

Listen. Listening conveys your sincere interest in the employee's job satisfaction and future development. By listening, you will increase your understanding of the employee and the PPDS will be more effective. Encourage the employee to open up and discuss the things she has on her mind that may be affecting her work. Often this kind of discussion produces reactions from the employee such as, *"This is the first time in two years that you've asked my viewpoint on things!"* This is common, and a good first step to a positively motivated employee and increasingly positive environment.

Be constructive, not destructive. Identify what needs to be improved and how to do it, don't just tell the employee how badly she has performed. Keep criticism impersonal by discussing job performance only and do not attack the person. For example, you could say, *"You are very irresponsible"* or you can say, *"This job was to be completed by Friday, the 12th, and it wasn't done until the 23rd."* The first statement is *opinion* and open to question and debate. The second is *fact*. The second statement is not putting the *person* in question, but rather her *behavior* or *actions*. This reduces the level of defensiveness and does not put the person's worth as an individual on the line.

Determine the cause of any poor performance and its solution. Encourage the employee to analyze any problem by asking, *"That's an unusual amount of billing errors...can you help me to understand what happened?"* Or, *"How can we prevent this from happening in the future."* Then wait for an answer.

Whenever a problem is identified (in a PPDS or otherwise), ask the employee for suggestions on how it can be improved, changed, eliminated, or resolved. This will help you build strong, concerned employees who are capable of thinking through issues to probable action or behavior that will result in a successful conclusion.

Make sure the solution is specific and set deadlines. If she is unable to come up with a solution at all, it is appropriate to make your own recommendations. If she comes up with a solution you feel is unacceptable, propose an alternate solution (one you feel is more appropriate) by saying, *"That's certainly one way of handling it; however, have you considered..."* and then continue on with your proposed solution.

Agree on a plan of action. Improvement in performance can only occur when both you and the employee perceive the problem from a similar perspective and both of you agree on the way to solve it. Put it in writing as an agreement between you and your employee. This kind of commitment gets better results than vague promises and serves as a benchmark against which progress can be measured. This will make your next PPDS much easier since you both know what is expected. This is also important documentation for grounds for dismissal, should this become necessary.

Discuss the employee's goals (over and above areas that need improvement) and where she is headed? What does she want to accomplish? Where is her next area for growth and development? Together, discuss these questions and determine how you can help her accomplish her objectives. Again, put these in writing.

Be inspirational. The employee should feel motivated to improve in a particular area or to stretch to new heights. She must feel that you believe in her, and that you believe she can tap more of her potential and reach new goals.

The PPDS Development Folder

A Personal and Professional Development Folder is best kept by both the employee and the doctor. This allows each person to have a complete picture of the employee's development process and history with the practice.

It should include several tabbed sections for easy information access. Here are a few suggestions, but you may think of other sections you would like to include.

- Employment data including application, resume, reference letters, W-4's, and salary history
- Job Description and Performance Standards
- A copy of each completed PPDS form (both the employee's and the doctor's)
- Training history (courses completed, including dental and related non-dental)
- Goals
- OSHA/Workman's Compensation/Medical Safety
- Miscellaneous

Summary of the PPDS

Personal and Professional Development Sessions are one of the highest-leveraged activities you can accomplish to stimulate, motivate and revitalize your employees and develop their talents. Too often they are left out of training and development programs, but they are an integral part of the process. Developing a PPDS program requires some groundwork and a job description is absolutely necessary against which you and the employee can measure performance. The time invested will pay great dividends for the employee, for you, and for your practice.

Chapter 16

MAXIMIZING EMPLOYEE POTENTIAL

The work ethic is still around, but in many situations it seems to be well hidden. Where are the employees who really want to work? Who really care about the practice? Who sincerely care about patients? Who want to be a true team member in every sense of the word?

People are becoming increasingly dissatisfied with the way their work is being organized and managed, and feel they are not receiving the rewards and recognition they expect. They don't feel a sense of belonging. At best, many feel like a disconnected piece of equipment that is plugged in at the beginning of the day, used, and then disconnected. At worst, they feel like an add-on piece of equipment patched into the end of the line or as a temporary addition to an ever changing parade of people.

Because of the increasing need for sensitivity to these issues, today's doctor must go beyond clinical skills, beyond the leadership and management skills, all the way to understanding human behavior.

Charlie, our nephew, is an extremely bright boy, but he did not do well in grade school and junior high. He didn't seem to get along *well with the teachers, received failing grades in many classes, and wasn't interested inparticipating in school activities such as sports.*

Just before Charlie's freshman year in high school my brother moved the family to a new town and different school district. My brother was assistant principal at the middle school nearby and therefore was involved with the faculty and staff. There seemed to be a new kind of spirit in this school district. The teachers seemed to go out of their way to give the students individual attention.

The result? Charlie's attitude changed dramatically. He liked his new teachers. He felt a part of the school. The teachers believed in him and he began to believe in himself. He became involved in school activities and team sports. And, first term grades averaged a 3.68 grade point, and have continued at this level in subsequent terms!

People want to do a good job, but we've got to believe in them and provide an atmosphere where their potential can come alive. Could it be that we haven't found the "right employees" because we haven't been the "right employer" or provided the "right atmosphere" for our employees to flourish? Are we disempowering our employees the way Charlie was disempowered?

Let's discuss a number of factors that affect morale and motivation, and identify ways to maximize our employees' potential.

Confrontation, Critique and Reprimand

Leadership requires the ability to positively confront the often difficult and always challenging personnel issues. When you do, you appeal to the highest standards and values of your team.

Often we don't want to confront because we are afraid of the response; we think we will be disliked or rejected, or feel the relationship will be damaged. Perhaps we feel the employee might quit. All these reasons for not confronting come from a position of fear.

When we hold something back that we are upset about or disappointed in we actually damage the relationship. *Since we communicate most what we think we are communicating least,* that which we hold back will appear non-verbally in the way we respond to a particular individual. Have you ever been unhappy or upset with an employee, didn't take the opportunity to speak with that employee about it directly, and then have that person come to you with, "Is something wrong?" or "Are you not feeling good?" or "Did I do something to make you mad?" All these are clear indications they are picking up on non-verbal communication.

People don't care how much you know until they
know how much you care.

When we have a true team, one that is committed to helping each other and the practice, we will have people who are willing to *speak* and to *listen*...regardless of what the communication is. This will never happen, however, until the doctor really cares about each of his or her team members as a person, and as an employee in the practice. There is no faking this concern.

Sincerity + Direction X Purpose = Results

Sincerity means true desire, belief and authenticity. It means being real. Direction is the focus you have. Purpose is your mission and vision. Your results will directly correlate to this equation, and how you live it out in your life.

Sometimes when we have an unusually talented individual technically we let other negative behaviors slide. It may be an attitude that isn't harmonious, negative comments or complaining, gossiping about other staff members, nit-picking or backbiting, unwillingness to fulfill responsibilities in certain areas, or an unwillingness to help or support other team members.

When we allow this type of behavior from any individual we cause the breakdown of the entire team. You probably will not see it immediately, but it will surface. It will begin happening underground at first; when it is bigger than is able to be repaired without leaving substantial scars, it will surface. There is no valid excuse for allowing any individual to stay on a team who is demonstrating disruptive, unacceptable, negative, or upsetting behavior. Any person in this category must be willing to correct the behavior. If the willingness isn't there or the change isn't forthcoming, that person must leave the practice if you want your practice to continue moving forward.

If the person in question indicates they want to make the change, be clear about your parameters and guidelines. Then, watch for the change. Watch to make sure the change is permanent and the individual doesn't slide back into old ways once the pressure is off. When you observe changed behavior, encourage it by positive comments and praise. If Mary Jane has not been supportive of a particular team member and you see that she has begun to go out of her way to say hello in the morning and talk with that person, commend her for it. Let her know you notice it. It is very disheartening to an employee who is sincerely willing to work at changing, to begin making the change and not have the boss notice.

Behavior that gets rewarded, gets repeated.

If, however, the change does not occur, it is time to find another team member. Too often a doctor (or manager) finds it easier to just put up with the situation and close their eyes to the disruption it is causing. Some even talk themselves into believing that it really doesn't make *that* much difference. But it does. Remember the old "one bad apple destroys the whole bunch" concept? It is true for your team also. The great employees with the good attitude and super work habits will be affected. It is up to you, as leader, to do something about the situation, confront it, and get it changed before it causes too much damage. Here are a few guidelines on how to positively confront an employees:

Always confront your employee in private. Never, never, never correct or reprimand an employee in front of another employee, a patient, or any other person. To do so loses you respect, credibility, and will cause the relationship to deteriorate so quickly you will wonder what happened.

Don't hold inventory. Don't save your reprimands, complaints and critiques until you can't hold them any longer, or dump them on the employee during a PPDS. This increases the anxiety level and creates the potential for an argument.

Don't smile. When you do, you will reduce your effectiveness in the point you are trying to make. Smiling suggests approval, and here you are speaking about something that doesn't meet your approval.

Describe the unacceptable behavior specifically. Be factual, not judgmental. Focus on behavior, not the person. In any confrontation, do not put the person's worth on the line. What is of concern is their behavior. If an employee feels you question her as a person, you will lose her trust and your ability to work with her effectively. Put the situation into perspective. The employee is not a bad person; that is not the issue. What is the issue is that the behavior or action was less than acceptable. Focus on performance and on solving problems, not on placing blame.

Not: Sue, I can't stand the way you handle patients.
But: Sue, the way you just handled Mrs. Jones does
     not go along with our values. Furthermore, it could
     lose us a patient, and an entire family. (Then go on to
     describe the behavior you witnessed)

Be specific. Tell the employee what she did wrong, specifically, based on what you observed and then tell her how it differs from your expectations. After a few moments of silence, encourage the employee to tell her side of the story, but don't allow excuses. Be open-ended with your question: *"In your opinion, Sue, how did this happen?"*

Honestly and openly listen to the employee's response. Is the employee making excuses or accepting responsibility? If the employee doesn't agree it is a problem, it won't be solved. Concern yourself with the *how*, the way it is said or done, but not the *why*. When we ask the why's or guess at the why's we put people on the defensive and it places us in a situation of making assumptions that may or may not be true.

Tell her how you feel about the behavior. Don't keep this inside. Let the employee know if you are angry or disappointed, but do it rationally without sarcasm, put-down or yelling.

Come to a mutual agreement. Both you and your employee must agree on the cause of the problem and the solution. Discuss how the situation can be changed, handled, or dealt with so it doesn't happen again in the future. Ask your employee for suggestions. If she doesn't have any, or you cannot go along with it, offer your suggestions. Then jointly agree on the most appropriate action.

Conclude by restating your employee's value to the practice. Let the employee know you feel she is an asset to your practice.

Once said, let it be. Don't repeat the reprimand or critique once you have expressed it clearly. Go back to work and let the employee know by your behavior that you are not "holding it against her," nor do you "feel indifferently" about her now.

Then, let the employee know that you will make a proper notation in her personnel file that you have had this discussion. If the issue is serious enough to warrant dismissal, write a warning memo to the employee briefly recapping the fact that you had the discussion and what behavior is expected, and put a copy in her file. If she improves or corrects the situation, write another memo indicating such and put a copy in her file once again. This effectively closes the subject.

If you want to have a strong practice, it requires strong employees working together. This requires that you nip in the bud any performance problems as soon as they are detected. If others see you tolerate this behavior, you will soon lose their respect and additional problems will be at your doorstep.

The issue of accountability is important here. Accountability is something we should all want to achieve in our practice...both with ourselves, as well as with our employees. The five principles of accountability are:

1. Accountability must begin with you in order for it to be effective.

2. If you do not hold others accountable, they *will not* and *cannot* reach their greatest potential.

3. If you do not hold others accountable, they will eventually lose respect for you.

4. Accountability must be consistent in order for it to be effective.

5. The psychological law of learning states that reinforced behaviors will most likely be repeated.

To reflect upon the accountability issue, ask yourself these related questions:

Am I being accountable as the leader?
How is this affecting the entire practice?
What can I do about it?
What am I *willing* to do about it?
Am I holding each team member accountable?
Are we being accountable as a team?

Unless it begins with us and we model the principle, we will most likely find accountability lagging in our employees.

Chapter 17

KEYS TO MOTIVATION

Today there are many dental offices competing for the limited supply of well-trained, motivated, and enthusiastic personnel. As a result, many dentists and practice managers are wondering what they can do to attract, motivate, and retain superior people.

Building morale and creating an atmosphere for motivating employees is part of your leadership role. The ability to do this increases as your skill in human relations and your ability to work effectively with your employees increases. Morale is a state of mind, an attitude, a point of view...and it colors the employee's feelings and influences her behavior in every aspect of her relationship with you, with her co-workers, with the practice and with her work.

Lack of understanding motivation, and therefore not following through on what it takes to create the atmosphere, leads to heavy turnover, ultimately increasing costs, and decreasing employee and patient satisfaction. Perhaps even worse than turnover is the disgruntled employee who does not leave the practice and remains, harboring resentment and withholding her commitment to the practice...and ultimately to the patients. Other symptoms where this atmosphere is missing is higher absenteeism, low morale, miscommunication and conflict.

Realize that all people are motivated. *Motivation means to be led from within by my beliefs, values and as a result, feelings and emotions.* When we say we want motivated employees what we really are saying is that we want people who have get up and go, are self starters, have a burning desire, knows where they are headed, etc. We want enthusiastic individuals who sincerely want to be in the practice.

Everything in this book is about motivation, but let's recap some of these factors that contribute to the positively motivated employee.

Provide a comfortable working environment, physically. Is your office bright and cheerful? Does it need some updating? Is it safe for the employees? Do they, and you, feel good about it? Have you ever asked your employees how they feel about it?

Be clear about values and ethics, and the practice culture. When employees know you stand for only the best, when they know you want to encourage them to become all they can be, when they know you care about them as individuals, they will feel great about working with you.

Get to know your employees. Identify their needs and find out what motivates them. This requires spending time with them to find out what they believe, what they want, where they are headed, and what fears or concerns they have relating to their work. Once you find out what they want, let them know you want to help them get it (as long as it does not go against your values, vision or mission). Then, help them find the methods or means of reaching those goals while also meeting the goals of the practice.

Tap the expertise and abilities of your employees. Involve them in planning whenever possible and appropriate. Have them, with you, brainstorm new and creative ways to be more effective, solve a problem, or resolve a conflict. Have them team up to help newer people in their areas of strength. Involving them helps gain commitment and establishes strong communication. When they feel involved it will have a positive impact on developing team spirit.

Ask for performance. Let your employees know what you expect and how you expect it to be completed. They want to know. They have no way of knowing what will be considered average, good or excellent performance unless you share your expectations with them. Don't keep them guessing.

Do not accept poor performance. If you do not let the employees know what they've done that you consider poor performance, it will most likely be repeated. And, in the process you will lose the respect, backing and enthusiasm of the other team members. Why should other team members give their all when someone on the team is doing nothing but creating problems, and is continually allowed to do it?

Provide feedback. Feedback is extremely important to each individual team member. It may be as simple as saying, *"Great job,"* or as complex as analyzing what was done and providing individualized prescriptive information.

Give lots of positive reinforcement. Praise your team in front of your patients regularly. Pass on compliments you receive from patients or suppliers *about* your team, *to* the team. Bring these up during morning huddles for a great way to start the day. Pass on some compliment or read the complimentary note you received in the mail. This builds your team and encourages more of the same great behavior.

You were great with Mrs. Smith.
You handled that difficult situation with Mr. Jones really well.
I noticed how you did (then identify what it is the employee is working on to improve that you just observed) and you're really making substantial improvement. Congratulations!"

When you praise, don't praise every little thing every time or it will quickly lose meaning. Praise can actually become a demotivator if the employees feels it is insincere. And, don't exaggerate.

Criticize the act or behavior when needed and appropriate, but not the person. State it clearly and in absolute terms. Don't leave it to your employees to "read" you or to "interpret" what you said. They may read you wrong. Give your employees all the information they need to improve performance, and as much as possible remain objective and free of personal bias.

Build relationships. Let your team members know you like them, respect them, and trust their intentions. If you don't, you'll create members on your team that will cause you problems no matter what. If you don't feel this way about a team member, it is best that the individual be allowed to find a position somewhere else where they can really grow and reach their potential. It will never happen if you don't feel good about the person.

Don't allow backbiting and gossip in your practice. Don't you do it, and don't allow other team members to do so. This principle must be carried out completely. Don't allow conversation to drift into tearing down other people, whether they are on your team or not, and present or not. If you allow yourself to be pulled into a conversation like this, it quickly raises questions in your employees mind about what you might say if they are not around. More important, it raises the question of your own integrity.

Thank your employees at the end of each day, for doing their part in making the day terrific. This lets them know they are really valued. Of course, you must be sincere when you give thanks.

Build a team and encourage a team spirit, a sense of belonging. Although many employees work rather independently, team spirit and a sense of belonging have been found to be two of the greatest determinants of motivation and high morale. In fact, employees often stay with an organization even if they could earn more somewhere else because a great psychological need is being met...the need to belong to and feel a part of the team.

Learn to see things from your team members point of view. This means listening and hearing them out before you give advice or direction.

Try to see beyond defensive behavior. Normally defensive behavior stems from insecurity due to a perceived threat or loss. Consciously or unconsciously we fight to protect our own good image of ourselves. It is easy to mistake a defensive reaction for resentment or resistance against ourselves when it is often an attempt by the other person to defend self-image. Try to offer understanding that will provide a safe and accepting climate for the employee to really express her true feelings and concerns without being made to look small or feel unworthy.

Model the behavior you want. Show by your actions what is important to you. This is one of aspect of leadership. Inspire confidence and motivate your employees by being consistent, sincere, considerate, and friendly. This doesn't mean you are out to win a popularity contest, but it does mean you treat your people with the same respect you want for yourself. People work best when they know what to expect from their doctor or supervisor, and that means being consistent and not guided by moods and whims.

Part of this is keeping your own motivation high. If you expect your employees to be enthusiastic, you must be enthusiastic first. If you are not enthusiastic your employees will waver in their commitment to your leadership and their enthusiasm will run low. Enthusiasm is contagious and a major factor in productivity....both yours and theirs.

Allow mistakes. Unless a person is making some mistakes, they're probably not doing very much growing. That is how we learn. Give your employees the unqualified understanding that you expect them to do what they do well, and to learn from the mistakes they make. Let them also know you understand that mistakes are a part of stretching and growing and you accept them. If you have employees always waiting for you to blow up over a mistake, you will always have employees who have one foot out the door.

Give your people opportunities to grow. (See chapter fourteen on training for many ideas here.)

Reward your team members for their contributions. There is nothing more demoralizing than to accomplish something at great expense (risking, stepping out of the comfort zone, doing something new they were afraid to try before, or simply putting in a great amount of time and energy on a particular project) and then not have the doctor or supervisor notice it. When an employee has shown progress or suggests a valuable idea, give credit to and praise her. When your team members are responsible for an idea you put into use in your practice, give them recognition for coming up with the idea. When you do, you will encourage them to continue contributing to the practice. Remember, what gets rewarded gets repeated. Employees like to feel they can contribute suggestions, and then be appreciated and recognized for them.

Help your people become and do their best. Use your PPDS to find out how you can help them. They will profit; you will profit by much happier, fulfilled, and therefore more productive employees; and in the long run, our entire society profits when people are encouraged to become their best.

Help them exercise self judgment in areas of their responsibility in the practice. This involves doing what needs to be done even if it means doing something a little differently than what is normally done. This is empowerment. Some people are uncomfortable with this because they feel an empowered employee might "give away the practice" or try to make a patient happy at the "expense of being profitable." But when an employee is empowered, they are also given what is necessary to know where those boundaries lie. If they are trained and truly empowered they will seldom handle situations in ways that will be negative for the practice.

Empowerment is a process that involves encouragement, consistency, partnership, values, and orientation in doing what is right and appropriate in a particular situation. The opposite is compliance or conformity, mandates coming down from on high on what to do in any situation, or doing what is easy, not necessarily what is right.

An empowered employee can strike a balance between his or her professional instinct and the policy and procedures of the practice. As a result, the patient relationship turns from a cold, superficial, "business only" contact into a warm, trusting and ongoing relationship.

Pay your people well for performance. Efficiency is important, as is effectiveness, and in our practices we must be concerned with both. Maybe you feel there is no "extra" to give beyond minimal compensation, but this becomes a chicken and egg issue. *There may well never be any extra until the people you have on your team feel they are getting a just wage, receiving recognition for a job well done and are paid according to the standard in the dental industry for your area.*

You say that's not the problem? That no matter how much you pay a particular employee they'll never be able to do much better? The question then to ask is, "Did I make a mistake of hiring the applicant who was willing to take the least amount of income?" If so, remind yourself that we usually get what we pay for.

Have fun. The team that can laugh together and enjoy each others company, both in the office and even outside, will stay together longer and accomplish much more than a team who does not. Too often we forget that "working for a living" can and should be fun. As the leader who establishes the pace in your practice, it is important you communicate to your team that having fun is not only okay, but really very important in creating a positive work environment. Fellowship is an important aspect in bringing fun to the workplace. Celebrating birthdays or anniversaries with lunch out, a cake, flowers, having the team get together for pizza after work, or gathering in someone's backyard for a barbecue, all lend an element of fun, enjoyment, and team spirit. Laugh a little! It's great for the soul and great for morale.

We strive to combine learning and fun in different ways in our practice. One time we all particularly enjoyed was when we scheduled an entire Wednesday afternoon for a team outing at the movie The Doctor . When we arrived at the theater we picked up the tab for lunch and/or goodies the team members wanted, as well as the movie. Since Norm and I had already seen the movie, and knew it could be a great introduction for discussing how our patients are greeted and treated, we also planned coffee and dessert at a local restaurant to follow. The movie was great and brought many feelings and emotions to the surface. This triggered a powerful discussion at the restaurant and ideas flowed freely. By the time we concluded the day, we had a deeper understanding of the patient, strong feelings about what we wanted to do for our patients, and a clearer understanding of each team member's responsibilities.

Another regular fun activity in our practice is that we take the entire staff out to lunch for a celebration of each employee's birthday. This is a fun time away where we discuss little, if any, work related topics.

During the summer months we have at least one barbecue at our home for our employees and their spouses, and we include the owner of the dental laboratory we use and his wife. At Christmas we always take these same individuals to dinner at a nice restaurant for a Christmas celebration.

It takes some thought to provide the little extras and have fun along the way. Ask your employees what they would like. Then begin to incorporate some fun activities into your practice. You'll get to know each other much better and the team will function more effectively. You might even decide to take your team to a practice management seminar in the Bahamas, Canary Islands, or Hawaii...who knows where...when your team is producing well. What a great thank you for work well done!

Keep your employees well informed. They want to know what is going on in the business and the industry. It is difficult to promote something you don't believe in, and you can't believe in something you know nothing about.

Celebrate your successes. When you have been working on a particular goal or an area of concern in the practice, and you have made some major growth, or if you have reached a particular goal...celebrate. Celebrating is one way of nourishing the spirit of the practice. Recognition, reward and celebration are ways of reaffirming to your team members that they are an important part of something significant, of something that really matters. Ask yourself: "Do your people do what they do with excellence. If not, why not?" I believe deep down most people want to, but it requires support and encouragement on your part. It means believing in them.

These several factors indicate that you, as leader, have a dynamic role. It is active, not passive. It takes work, time, and attention, but the rewards are far greater than the effort expended. Not only do you benefit, but so do your employees. They become happier, more productive, and more fulfilled. Certainly the first benefactor, and the one that impacts the practice the most, is your patients. They will love to come to your office. They will sense the team spirit, the camaraderie, the caring and the concern you feel for each other. And with this, they will feel well taken care of, and want to return again and again. Further, your family and the employee's family will benefit. It is impossible to feel good about what you do and the time you invest doing it and not feel better about everything else in your life. And as a result of happier, more fulfilled people, our world will be a better place.

Recently I was giving an inspirational keynote presentation to stimulate the participants to think bigger...to develop a deeper understanding and belief that they are more than they currently consciously realize.

Prior to speaking I was standing by the table filled with my books and tapes, greeting people as they entered. One particularly beautiful woman caught my eye as she was looking through one of the books. I leaned over to her and said, "You have absolutely beautiful hair." (It was coal black, shiny and flowed to her waist). Without looking up, she mumbled under her breath something barely audible. I thought for a moment and then leaned over to her again and said, "Excuse me, did you just say that's all you have?" And she replied, "Yes."

I moved a little closer and whispered, "I am so happy you are here tonight, because that's exactly what I will be addressing. You have so much more than just your hair."

After the presentation this woman waited while several others approached me to speak. When her turn came she moved forward confidently, with the most beautiful smile on her face. She was glowing! And she said, "You have just given me a gift you'll never understand. I feel as though maybe I do have more than my hair...and I do have a dream... and I am going to make it come true." She went on, "When I see you again, some time in the future, I'll come up and tell you what I have become and have been able to accomplish."

What most people need is someone to believe in them...and someone who can show them what the tools are and how they can be used to make happen whatever it is they want to accomplish. Be sure your people have the tools, the time, the information, and adequate training.

We all want productive practices, and productivity, in the end, depends upon two things:

1. Motivation. Arousing and maintaining the "will to work" effectively means having committed team members, not just those who work because they are coerced to work.

2. Rewards. Effective performance is recognized and rewarded in terms meaningful to the individual, whether it be financial, psychological or both.

All the areas identified above fall into one or both categories. Anthony Robbins says that we do what we do for one of two reasons: To avoid pain or to increase pleasure. You do it, and your employees do it. It's up to the leader to provide an atmosphere that includes both...and that's a motivating environment!

We are responsible for the quality of our relationships and the quality of our responses. Every interaction with our employees, as with our patients, is a moment of truth. As a reflection for what we've just covered, write down each team member's name and ask yourself the following questions about each:

What could I do that would improve the quality of this relationship?
How can I be a better leader where this person is concerned?
How can I encourage/empower this person to be the best she can be?

Expectations as Self-Fulfilling Prophecy

Much of what happens in your practice depends upon your expectations. What you believe becomes a self-fulfilling prophecy.

The doctor who sincerely believes he or she is successful and productive can motivate employees to follow the lead. If you believe an employee has no chance for success, it will most likely become a self-fulfilling prophecy. On the other hand, if you do believe in the employee and communicate these expectations, that too will most likely become a self-fulfilling prophecy.

Your positive expectations, however, must pass the test of reality before they can be translated into performance. Employees will not be motivated to grow and reach higher levels of effectiveness or productivity unless they consider the expectations realistic and achievable. If they are encouraged to strive for unattainable goals, or goals they *feel* are unattainable, they will eventually give up trying and settle for less than they are truly capable of achieving.

Putting the "Heart" in Employee Development

The human side, the heart side of employee development doesn't necessarily mean just what you do. How you give of yourself and your attitude has a strong impact on your employees and their success. Regardless of what we have believed about the bell curve in years gone by, the majority of employees you hire will be successful, mediocre, or fail depending upon your care and feeding of them. They must be supervised and evaluated, but it is how you do it that makes the difference.

Sometimes you may be called upon just to listen to an employee who is having difficulty or facing some problem or crisis in their personal life. Listen and let her know you care. You don't have to have all the answers or be a licensed psychologist to let her know you care and are willing to listen.

Take the time to let your people know personally that you appreciate the job they have done and are doing. As mentioned earlier, take a few minutes at the end of the day to thank them for their contribution to the team. Go out of your way once in a while. That's all part of giving of yourself. It doesn't take much time, but it really builds morale and team spirit.

Finally, integrity and trust provide an atmosphere where employees can develop and produce optimal results. In this atmosphere, where people are treated as human beings with dreams, expectations, and goals, and when they know it is sincere and not an attempt at manipulation, they will gladly give the second effort...indeed a third, a fourth and even more.

When you make the heart connection in management you will receive one of the greatest rewards possible: you will see the person you brought into your practice grow and succeed. This kind of success can't be measured in dollars, but brings with it incredible satisfaction and fulfillment.

Chapter 18

TERMINATING EMPLOYEES

When you work with your employees and give them continual feedback, you will find that the same procedures that help most employees grow and develop greater skills will also reveal those who cannot or choose not to grow in your environment. This on-going evaluation prevents employees from being able to hide behind past performance. It becomes clear who should move out of the practice and on to another opportunity. Any conclusion for dismissal isn't the *boss* deciding the employee was incompetent or inadequate. Rather, the *employee* will also see the poor fit between her talents and efforts and what the job requires.

The most humane way to work with employees who are not as productive as you feel they should be is to attempt to save them as soon as you recognize the deficiency, and long before dismissal becomes inevitable. You owe it to the people you bring on board to try and help them work up to your expectations and their capacity. Otherwise, you may feel guilty and find it even more difficult to terminate them if they don't work out.

Guilt feelings sometimes stem from unrealistic expectations at the time of employment (by the doctor or supervisor) that no employee could ever live up to. Another reason for guilt, however, is that little things that should have been corrected at the time they happened were overlooked or dismissed. Later it becomes difficult to reconcile all these "little things" without the employee feeling "dumped" on. Situations like these often increase the guilt of doctors or supervisors because they know they played a significant part in the employee's failure by neglecting to do what needed to be done at the time.

An example of this happened to one of my client's. This particular doctor had a very difficult time confronting employees with problem areas. One of his employees was creating dissension in the practice among other employees. This employee had been with the practice a year or so and seemed to be very positive when she was hired. She did a great job clinically as an assistant. Nevertheless something had changed and she was not positive, didn't work with the other team members as a team, and griped and complained behind the doctor's back to other employees and patients.

Even though one of the other employees, who was not one to gossip or be negative, repeatedly expressed her concern, the doctor avoided the issue. The difficult employee was "fudging" on her time card, even to the extent of including days she didn't actually work! She and another employee were continually huddled in a corner somewhere talking quietly... and when anyone would approach them they would immediately stop. She also discussed all her problems (her husband, finances, children, etc.) with the patients. Nevertheless, the doctor tried to deny that it was necessary to take action.

Finally, when things were so bad the situation couldn't be ignored, the employee was approached by the doctor. One discussion didn't calm the rage nor clear the situation. The end came when the employee quit (first making a few threats) and walked out yelling at the doctor.

It is most interesting to note that during one of the final discussions the employee said to the doctor, "Why didn't you bring these things up when they first bothered you so we could have dealt with them then, and it wouldn't have had to come to this."

Good question. The moral of this story: Don't wait. When you see something that is not working, when you don't like behaviors taking place in your practice, don't delay in bringing them to the attention of the individual involved. Perhaps the employee above could have been saved. Perhaps not. The answer will never be known. But this much is clear, there's no way the situation could be salvaged by *not* dealing with it.

When an employee is terminated for performance that is not up to standards, it should not come as a surprise. Too often, however, it does. I have seen situations where an employee has been given a satisfactory performance rating on an evaluation just because it was easier than confrontation. When an employee does not meet the expected standards of performance, the doctor should not wait until the final termination interview to discuss the problem. This is not fair to the employee, the doctor, the other employees, the patients, or the practice as a whole. By being candid, honest, and open, you give an employee the opportunity to improve. When an area that needs improvement is discussed, the employee will not be surprised later if termination results because improvement was not forthcoming. Whenever we postpone or try to avoid unpleasantries, they almost always worsen over time.

Dismissal, however, should only occur after the failure of genuine efforts to help the employee succeed. When it has been determined that termination is the only reasonable course of action left, then some fundamental guidelines should be followed in approaching the dismissal.

First, be prepared. Terminating an employee is a significant management responsibility. It should always be preceded by careful fact gathering, analysis and decision making. All you have done in the process of trying to build the employee to acceptable levels of performance should already be documented in the employee's development folder.

Second, prepare the explanation. The logic for termination should be clarified and justified in advance of the exit interview. If the employee is being discharged due to budgetary reasons, financial data should show why the company must take this action. If an employee is being fired for poor performance, her record should justify the action. The explanation to the employee must show that the decision was inevitable, that there was no acceptable alternative based on the circumstances. This should be very clear to the employee already if you have done your job in discussing performance along the way.

Third, communicate the finality. The objective of the termination interview is to communicate to the employee the decision for termination, to state clearly the reasons, and to let the employee know the decision is final.

Fourth, even though the decision is final, the employee should be given an opportunity to discuss the reasons if she so desires. Obviously with the previous discussion this should be clear, but if it isn't, do provide time for discussion.

Terminating an employee is an unpleasant part of your work, and one of the major sources of anxiety for doctors, managers, and supervisors in all businesses. Simply the thought of it creates distress for many! Nevertheless, it is part of your job and should be done just as efficiently as you would any other important practice function.

When unpleasant tasks come before you as the leader, they should be confronted with thoughtfulness, care and authority...but they should be confronted. Walking away from them, ignoring them in the hope they will disappear by themselves, or postponing action in anticipation of a miracle will only result in further distress, lowered morale among all team members, and decreased productivity. Additionally, patients will pick up on the dissatisfaction and your image will suffer.

Exit Interviews

When an employee has not been terminated by you, but has made the decision to leave herself, an exit interview can provide a wealth of information. Let the departing employee know the interview is confidential, unless there are legal issues involved, and tell her why you are doing the interview (to continually improve the practice). Ask for her responses to these questions: *How would you, or what what you do to, improve the practice? If you could change anything, what would it be?* Then, carefully examine the responses and use the information to make changes where appropriate.

> **Note:**
> Our society is rapidly changing and with it, termination laws. It is important that you refer to specific procedures and guidelines established by state and federal laws.
> The above are general guidelines and form the basis for termination, but should not be considered all inclusive.

Chapter 19

TEAM MEETINGS

People have gotten together to exchange information long before the beginning of recorded history. And today the need for meetings continues. Whether to develop new approaches or evaluate existing processes and programs, well run meetings get the team involved, working together, and moving in the same direction.

Meetings are formal and informal, planned and impromptu. Some are special, some are on-going. Meetings are very important and necessary to the success of organized effort. It is often in conference that ideas are exchanged and developed, vital information communicated and shared, and decisions reached that dramatically impact the practice.

A meeting should be planned and conducted to communicate the most constructive and meaningful information in the shortest time possible. Simply because people have been called together does not mean that anything of value to the team will be accomplished unless some preparatory work is completed.

Identify the Need

Know why you are having a meeting. Meetings need to be purposefully directed in order to be effective in time, money and results. Before scheduling the meeting, consider whether or not something worthwhile can actually be accomplished by gathering your people together. If so, establish that purpose clearly. Some reasons for having a meeting include:

- problem solving
- decision making
- instructing or training
- motivating
- planning
- reporting or informing

A meeting should be planned and conducted so as to impart the most constructive and meaningful information in the shortest possible time.

Guidelines for Effective Meetings

Some practices steer clear of meetings as much as possible because of the cost involved due to lost production, as well as the salaries or hourly wages paid for the time of the meeting. Nevertheless, meetings are often underutilized as an opportunity in dentistry to build the team. Meetings, properly planned and conducted, are an excellent way for participants to seek a shared understanding of issues, problems, and conflicts, and then cooperate in identifying how to solve them for the good of all involved, as well as the good of the practice.

While particular kinds of meetings have various and unique considerations, there are some general rules that apply to all types of meetings. Using these ensures the elimination of countless wasted minutes and hours, and substantially increases the effectiveness of any meeting.

Know the purpose. Where does it fit in? Why are you calling the meeting? Think "reason" first, "meeting" second.

Set goals for the meeting. What do you want to accomplish? How will you know it has happened?

Make sure the appropriate participants are in attendance.

*Select an appropriate location for the meeting...*and arrange for no phone calls to be placed or received during the meeting.

Choose an appropriate time. It is difficult to schedule meetings in the evening after normal hours, or at lunch time. People need the lunch break for errands, to recharge, to make phone calls, eat lunch, etc. At the end of the day people are usually tired and want to get home to attend to family affairs. They won't be as fresh and able to give their best focus and attention, or generate ideas and creative solutions the same as they would in the morning or earlier afternoon.

Prepare an agenda and inform everyone adequately of the purpose. Even for impromptu or informal meetings it is a good idea to put in writing the focus of the meeting and any particulars in order to stay on track. If you want the team members to suggest items for the agenda, ask early for their items so they can be worked into the agenda. If possible, give the agenda to the team members ahead of time so they can review it, and be ready for discussion.

Let the participants know what "homework" is to be completed before the meeting. If you would like someone to prepare a presentation, or if they are to come ready to discuss an issue, let them know in advance. If you want them to read an article for discussion, again make sure they have it far enough in advance.

Bring whatever you need for the meeting to the meeting. This includes communication tools, projectors, flip charts, screens, charts, markers, tape recorder, statistics, etc.

Begin the meeting on time.

Begin with an ice-breaker to warm up the team. You could begin by having each person tell something about themselves, perhaps something non-work related that others don't know about them. Or have them tell one good thing that has happened personally since the last time you met. Maybe you'll want to have each person share one great thing that happened in the practice in the last week.

The ice breaker is simply that...to give the meeting a jump-start and get the team involved and interacting with each other. Don't spend much time here. Limit each person's response to a minute or two, or whatever you feel is reasonable.

Keep the meeting on target. Follow the agenda as closely as possible; consider time limiting the agenda items.

Use visual aids for greater impact. The more we involve the visual, auditory, and kinesthetic in our meetings, the better chance we will have to reach our people. We have different learning styles and some people learn better by *seeing*, others by *hearing*, and some find it difficult to learn at all unless they can *do* whatever it is.

Encourage participation. Effectiveness of the meetings will be in direct proportion to the participation of the team members.

Record important points or follow-up steps or procedures. Announce what has been accomplished, who is responsible to take the next step(s) and identify any unresolved questions?

Accountability comes into play here. Whoever is leading the meeting should make sure that everyone heard the same thing and are in agreement as to what decisions were made and what they mean.

When you make decisions and gather information in the meeting, be sure to put those decisions into action. Set a timetable and make it happen. Information without implementation leads to depression.

Bring closure to the meeting. Thank the participants for their input and work accomplished. If desired, allow some time for the participants to briefly reflect on the success of the meeting.

Essentially, all these points stress a very important factor...organization. With a bit of planning, and participation from all involved, meetings can be productive, motivating, and a source of valuable information and communication.

Types of Meetings

In the dental practice, there are a few common types of meetings that are of value. Here are a few of the most common, and most effective:

Morning Huddle. The morning huddle is an invaluable tool for your practice. It can alleviate a great deal of stress that might normally result without it. It will actually increase productivity if it is well engineered. The emotional tone of the day is set by you, the leader, and it is your attitude at the beginning of the day, in the huddle, that will determine how the rest of the day will proceed.

Just as a builder wouldn't begin building a house without a blueprint, nor the wise pilot take off without his flight plan, neither is it a good idea for you to begin your day without a huddle. This is your blueprint for the day.

The morning huddle accomplishes the following:

- Helps each team member make the transition from their personal life to their professional life
- Sets the tone for the day
- Saves time throughout the day by cutting down on mistakes
- Allows a planned approach to patient treatment
- Allows the team to operate as a team and begin the day in harmony

Some of the more common huddle activities are:

- The receptionist gives input on patient flow or new patient referrals, as well as offers pertinent information regarding new or returning patients (such as the new patient is extremely afraid of injections, or Mrs. Jones just returned from Hawaii for two weeks, or Susie Smith just had a baby, etc.). She may indicate which patients were unable to be confirmed (and therefore are potential no-shows), or who needs attention from a financial arrangement standpoint.

- Confirm that lab work is back for patients coming in. Actually, this should be checked at least a day or two before, and just reconfirmed in the huddle.
- Hygiene patients are reviewed for periodontal therapy needs and the need for radiographs.
- Check for any patients with diagnosed treatment that is not completed, and work towards getting them scheduled.
- The dental assistant is given instructions on particular dental procedures or materials needed, and particular needs for an individual patient such as operatory or set-up is identified.
- Check for consistency of treatment...that is, be aware of patients you need to follow-up with concerning recommended treatment or home care instructions (such as Peridex rinses, etc.)
- Prepare common objectives or important points you want to get across to a particular patient.
- Allow time for "check-in" by each of the team members. How are each of them feeling today?
- Briefly recall what your goals are for the day.
- Visualize. At the end of the huddle, have everyone close their eyes and visualize what kind of day you want it to be. Perhaps lead them through a visualization with some thing like:

For just a moment, see the day before you. In your mind, see the patients smiling as they approach the office. They like the experience of being here with us and they are actually looking forward to coming. See each of us working together as a team harmoniously...helping and supporting each other emotionally, and well as with tasks that need to be accomplished. Notice how the patients are ready and willing to pay for their services upon their departure. See how easily our patients accept the proposed treatment and schedule their next appointment. Notice, too, that everyone is on time for their appointments and how easily we stay on track.

Take your own pulse now...it is the end of the day. Observe how good you feel...how energized you are because we worked so well together and with our patients.

Now, take this with you as we begin our day and draw all this to yourself ..and more.

Visualizations are powerful. By beginning your day with a clear, positive focus, you can actually give yourself a jump-start on the kind of day you want.

We draw to us that which we focus on.

At the beginning or end of the huddle, it might be a good idea to have one or two people walk through the office and look at the practice through the eyes of the patients. Is everything in place? Is the reception area clean and organized? Are any lights out, magazines torn or outdated that need to be removed, etc.

A well thought out huddle will ensure that you can move into your day stress-free, organized, and ready to enjoy working with your patients and each team member.

Practice Check-up Meetings. These are meetings to communicate the health of the practice. Here is where you discuss the number of new patients; accounts receivable balance; productivity; collections (and the percentage); treatment plans presented vs. treatment plans accepted; broken, canceled and changed appointments; practice expenses; and anything else necessary to know where the practice stands and where you are in relation to your goals.

Some doctors don't feel comfortable sharing this information with the team, but it is important to realize that just as with any sports team, people don't usually enjoy playing the game if they don't know the score as they go along. Sharing and discussing with the team helps them to "belong." It also helps them develop ownership in the practice. When they do, they'll go the extra mile to accomplish the vision, mission and goals of the practice.

Vital Statistics of the Team Meetings. These are meetings to determine the effectiveness of the team itself. Here is where we learn how we can better help each other. Perhaps for this meeting you would want to make a list of the weaknesses that are hampering the growth of the team and the practice. This can be done during the meeting itself with all team members giving input. Another approach is to have each person write comments before the meeting, then have them compiled and put in writing. The input is then used to discuss ways you can improve. Ask other questions, too. *How can we better help each other? What are some habits of team members that hinder greater teamwork and commitment?* This kind of direct question is best handled in a team where trust has been developed and the team functions well as a team. *Are there any complaints?*

Whatever these comments or questions produce, the following four guidelines will help you deal with them effectively.

1. *Discuss the input and turn it into a goal.* What would the positive statement be (the corollary of the problem)?

   For example, someone says: "The instruments are not being kept up and patients are having to wait longer than necessary to be seated."

   Turn it into a goal statement:
   Not: Don't keep patients waiting because instruments are not yet sterilized.

   But: Instrument sterilization follows a process that allows us to keep ahead of our needs and get patients seated immediately.

2. *Identify what you feel needs to happen in order to achieve it.*

3. *Determine how you will measure progress and how often.* Know what it will "look like" once it is achieved.

4. *Establish an expected date for accomplishment.*

Achieving the Next Level Meetings. Here the entire team meets for a full day or two to express their ideas of how to achieve the next level in the practice. First, of course, there needs to be clarification of what the next level is and agreement reached. Then, the time is spent in identifying what it will take, how you will go about it, what is the timeline, who is responsible for what, and any other pertinent factors. Two days work well because it allows team members time to digest what happened the first day and ponder what was discussed, and return the next day even more charged up. Scheduling shorter follow-up sessions at appropriate time intervals following this type of meeting is helpful to determine where you are on your plan (such as 3 or 6 months later). This kind of meeting is often accomplished in a retreat type setting.

Practice Retreats. This is a longer meeting, but it is still a meeting. Retreats may be one day, or several. Usually they involve scheduled time and free time. The bottom line to a retreat, however, is that it allows some uninterrupted time for the team to function as a team, make decisions, and work towards practice objectives. Anything you feel is worthy of your time and discussion can be the topic of the retreat.

Some of the more common topics, however, include development of a new or refined vision or mission statement, clarification of values, or training in a particular area.

Retreats typically are held away from the practice, whether it be in the same city or perhaps at a distant location. Options include retreat centers, mountain cabins, a house by the ocean, or some other appropriate spot. One key to a successful retreat is being away with no telephone interruptions, no thought of getting back to the office to check on this or that, and having the ability to focus totally on the subject at hand. Usually the dress is casual and people feel comfortable in letting their hair down, taking off their "professional title" and being together as equals on a mission that is productive and fun.

Often it is helpful to have a facilitator conduct your retreat so no one individual is the leader in this environment. The facilitator should work with the doctor to clearly identify the purpose of the retreat. The facilitator should then be able to plan the retreat so the team and practice objectives are met.

Whatever the purpose of the meeting, be sure it is well thought out and planned. With careful attention to a few key principles, effective meetings can bring the team together and stimulate bonding that is so essential to the dental practice team.

Chapter 20

TEAM BUILDING

Just as on any ball team, whether it be basketball, baseball, football, soccer or any other sport, the team is the key to winning. Without the team working together as a team, the chances of winning are pretty slim. The same is true of your dental team. All members must work together as a team in order to be effective and to accomplish the practice goals, live the mission, and strive for the vision. It is important to understand that just because people come together as a work group does not mean they will work as a team.

How about your practice. Do you have a *group* of people working together? Or do you have a *team?* Teamwork is more than just desirable...it is a necessity for the kind of practice most of us would like to have. When a team truly exists, team members *love* their work, love to *go* to work and they *want* to go to work. Novel concept? But it's true!

> The basic role of the leader is to foster mutual respect
> and to build a complementary team,
> where each strength is made productive,
> and each weakness is irrelevant.
> *Dr. Stephen Covey*

As discussed earlier, it is important to interview, select and hire, then train, organize, and motivate each member of the team for maximum performance. We also discussed the importance of your vision and mission...and communicating that with passion to the team. Just as in sports, every team begins with a game plan. You, too, must have one for your people. Leadership is extremely important here, and it comes strongly into play from the beginning. If an employee gets off to a bad start it may dictate the direction of his or her development...and on a downhill basis. As with a professional ball team, the so so's don't often hang around for a second season.

Identifiers of a Team

There are five identifiers basic to a team. The first is that a team is **synergistic**. The acronym TEAM stands for:

Together Everyone Accomplishes More.

The total accomplished is greater than the sum of what could be accomplished individually. A team is **interdependent.** The members of the team depend upon and trust each other to carry out his or her responsibilities. Each person supports the others. If one member of the team succeeds, all succeed. If one member of a team fails, the entire team falls short. A team must also be **stimulating,** that is, the action and attitude of the members spur the team on to achievement...often beyond what one feels was his or her personal ability. Without stimulation the members of the team will lose interest, become bored and production will decrease. A team must also be **enjoyable.** The members must like working together and feel a sense of belonging. They must find the work environment pleasurable and receive personal satisfaction from the work they do. There must be an element of fun in the workplace. Finally, the team must be **civilized**. The individual members must be courteous, diplomatic, civil, and in spite of personality differences, willing to interact and share.

When any one of these components is missing the team is less than it could be. It loses its' "teamness" and becomes simply a group of people working together. And, where teamwork is missing in a practice, you will most likely find morale problems.

are the important characteristics of each *individual* to be an effective *team member.*

Characteristics of an Effective Team Member

Each person requires feedback and is required to give feedback. Trust must exist within the team, however, in order for this to occur. Each person must be trustworthy and willing to trust. Positive feedback is important for every person for their contribution to the team. It is helpful to remember that positive feedback is both commending what was done that was great...as well as communicating in a positive, constructive way those things that are not acceptable or up to the team standards.

> It is good to remember in giving feedback that judgment is weakness, and observation is wisdom.

Each individual must understand the impact he or she has on others in the team. Since we don't operate in a vacuum, and we must work interdependently, attitudes and behaviors will affect everyone else on the team.

Each must help identify and resolve problems, and acknowledge issues and concerns that are affecting the team and the entire practice. Every person has an active role in the practice. It shouldn't be left entirely to the office manager or doctor to identify areas in need of improvement, reworking, restructuring, or change.

Each individual must be willing to take ownership, and willingly and positively confront when the situation calls for it. This requires developing good interpersonal skills, and the ability to confront behavior and not the person. Most people today are no longer willing to be told what to do and simply do as they are told. The key to a top performing staff is to have a team that feels good and feels valuable. It's up to you, the leader, to generate those feelings in yourself and in your staff. One way is to hold each person accountable for themselves individually and as a team member.

It is important to reiterate here that team members must allow mistakes in order to grow, and to learn from mistakes when they are made. People who are not willing or seem incapable of accepting mistakes as a part of the learning and growing process do not belong on the team. It takes only one team member to be out of alignment with the rest of the team to destroy the team's effectiveness.

Each must encourage others to communicate and participate. Employees like to be asked what they think as long as the person asking is sincere about wanting the feedback. Once again, if the team members are not working toward the same mission, the feedback is meaningless and will eventually lead to the deterioration of the team and individuals leaving the practice. A successful team can flourish in an environment where all team members feel they can contribute and communicate openly. Sometimes, however, because of personality or past experience, certain individuals will be fearful of making a suggestion or expressing feelings. It is up to every member of the team to create an environment that is conducive to openness and encourages responsiveness from other team members.

Each must be willing to offer assistance, when time is available, to another team member who is in need or overloaded.

No matter how talented a member of your team is individually, unless he or she is willing to work together with everyone else on the team, the team and its results will suffer.

There are several human tendencies developed and reinforced throughout our lives. Many people believe they don't measure up to others, so they compare their lives to others. As a result we tend to put ourselves down with unwarranted assumptions. We tend to resist change. We prefer to think our own thoughts and we sometimes listen selectively, hearing only what we want to hear. We sometimes force people into situations instead of creating an environment where they can blossom and grow. We like choices; the feeling that we have no choice creates reactive responses rather than proactive response. And finally, the mind's natural negative alignment causes many people to think or believe that miracles, goals, plans, and dreams will not come true.

These are all human tendencies we must be aware of as we

much more beautiful and there will be sunshine along the way. And when the rainclouds hit, as they sometimes will, there will still be the hope that the vision holds lighting our way, and a rainbow to remind us that the hope is real.

We've come full circle. A team doesn't happen by chance. It must be developed and worked at. A team is much like a family or any other relationship. Unless we take the time to nurture it, it will plateau and then begin to wither. Unless we take the time to get to know the members involved, the relationships will be superficial and the sense of belonging will be missing. Unless we invest the necessary effort we will get just what we have earned...not much less, and certainly not much more.

Chapter 21

COMPENSATION

Compensating people is an important functional element of the practice, yet intense debate and mystery often surround it. There is probably more division of thought on this than on any other management activity. Nevertheless, attracting, motivating and retaining personnel is an essential element in creating and maintaining an effective, successful practice. This is the underlying precept of the compensation package. When we consider compensation we can use the equation:

$$\text{Monetary payoff} + \text{Psychic Payoff} = \text{Total Compensation}$$

We've said that behavior that gets rewarded gets repeated. But let's not confuse what this really means. People like money, yes. But money isn't the only thing that is important or the only factor in compensation. In fact, money itself is not a motivator. Once a raise is received it is quickly absorbed into the budget as *necessary* money (it is no longer *extra*), and the employee is looking forward to the next raise. This happens because we perpetuate it! We don't have to hand out salary increases on an annual or semi-annual basis just because an employee is still with us. There are many

sphere promotes a healthy sense of autonomy, contentment, and satisfaction in the work done.

Similarly, my belief based on working with hundreds of corporations and practices, is that *if any bonus is instituted* it should promote teamwork, cooperation, coordination, innovation, and creativity. It should focus and concentrate efforts on the common goal rather than on some personal, individual goal. These are the keys to practice success and are the elements to be considered in designing any bonus program.

Objective goals under the direct control of the individual, upon occasion, may be appropriate. This individual system is best when the employee's own actions directly control results; i.e., increased efforts increase productivity. There are disadvantages to this individualized system, however, because it focuses on the individual effort, decreases cooperation and often generates competition, divisiveness and hard feelings among employees.

Bonuses and salary increases are primarily an *extrinsic* reward system. The reward comes from *outside* the employee, contrasted with an *intrinsic* reward system in which the employee is rewarded by a feeling of achievement, responsibility and meaningful contribution to the practice.

If you remain committed to a bonus system, there are a couple factors that should be taken into consideration. A bonus program should be *extra pay for extra effort,* not pay for doing the normal job. It must be clearly understood by the employees and able to be objectively calculated. It is also important to understand that the doctor must have a giving spirit to make the bonus system work. If the bonus is continually held over the heads of the employees as "see how good you have it here, " or "don't you understand just how much I am doing for you" it can backfire and create very unhappy, unhealthy feelings in the team members toward you, their work and the practice. A bonus program must come from your heart. It must be something you really feel good about giving. And your employees must be able to feel that sincerely. If these criteria are not met the program may generate frustration, poor morale, and actually *reduce* performance.

Key to making any bonus program work is setting the standards for the bonus program. If the requirement or goal necessary to achieve is considered too high to be achievable, it will decrease morale. If the goal is set too low it won't generate enthusiasm. The same is true of the reward. If the rewards are too low, employees will not feel the excitement and enthusiasm toward reaching the goal. If the reward is too high, however, and you must subsequently lower it, it will be negatively perceived by the team. Better to start lower with the rewards and build to a comfortable level, but well within reason.

Here's an example of a bonus opportunity that won't become expected or a "regular." And rather than put the burden on the doctor to come up with the entire bonus, each member of the team has a big part in making the bonus happen. Let's say a cruise has been announced for your dental team. The cost is $1,500 per person, double occupancy. You and your staff are enthusiastic about the location of the cruise, the pampering while on board ship, and the relaxation and recreation time away from the home front. You say you can't afford $1,500 per person for each of your staff members and you and your spouse as well? You don't have to. Here's where the team effort comes in.

Gather your team together. Enthusiastically present the cruise idea to the team. Create a visual picture and let them know what's in it for them. Then say, "Does this sound like something we'd all like to do?" If you've got a resounding yes, then throw out the challenge. "The cost of the cruise will be $1,500 per person. Now...we've got x number of months until the sailing date. How can we generate this kind of additional income to cover the cost of the cruise for us all?" Then brainstorm how you can generate the revenue together. There are many possibilities here. Perhaps you will all decide to work an additional hour a week seeing patients in the practice, and everyone does this without salary for that hour. The profits generated by that hour are then placed in a "kitty" so to speak (the bank) and left to build toward the funds needed. If you know about the cruise 7 months in advance and you have 26 working weeks (therefore 26 hours) and your profits are 45% for that hour and you average a $450 production hour (including the hygienist)...that's $247.50 net times 26 weeks or $6,435.00 in the kitty toward the cruise. That would cover the cost of 4.29 people for the cruise. If you are in a practice with one hygienist, one front desk person and one assistant, you've not only covered all the employees but yourself as well!

penses within the parameters of a financially healthy practice.

You may feel you can't afford to provide more than minimal salaries and few benefits, but you can't afford not to either. What you save by not providing good salaries or hourly wage and benefits, is really a drop in the bucket compared to what you can produce when you have motivated, committed, happy employees. And you'll never have this kind of employee until they first know you care about them.

Whatever benefits you offer, make sure your employees understand their benefits, and what they are worth (in dollars). Unless they know, they cannot appreciate what you are providing for them.

Part Three

*You and Your Patients:
Building the Practice*

Chapter 22

MARKETING

Marketing is positioning you and your practice in the minds of your patients. It is, very simply, making your mark.

> Positioning is not what you do to a product or service,
> but it is what you do with that product or service
> in the mind of the patient.

It is the positioning of your practice that will determine your success. Positioning requires understanding your practice identity, what you really want your practice to look like, and then communicating that identity to prospective patients.

Many people think of paid advertising when they think of marketing...but it is much broader than this. Whether or not you invest any funds in marketing, it is important to understand at the outset that everything you do and say, and everything your team members do and say, is also marketing. Every single one of you is an ambassador for the practice. When we understand it this way, we can see the tremendous marketing that goes on day in and day out, whether we have recognized it as such or not. Because marketing is dynamic, not static, it is a vital, essential function of a successful dental practice.

Perhaps you're thinking that marketing isn't something you need in your practice. Maybe you have a full practice and don't feel the need for new patients to come through your door. There are few practices, if any, in a position where no new patients are needed. Patients die, move, complete major treatment and are basically on maintenance, so new patients are always needed. Although your financial investment in marketing can be minimal, it is still an investment that must be made. A practice in this situation is similar to a patient who needs only routine preventive dental care. This person doesn't need any in-depth treatment, but to keep them in that condition they still need regular continuing preventive care...both at home and with regular visits to your office.

Some believe marketing has only to do with attracting new patients. Actually, marketing also has to do with maintaining the patients you already have in your practice. This, perhaps even more than attracting new patients, is the biggest reason to understand marketing and how it is affecting your practice minute by minute, day by day, month by month, and year by year.

Marketing is patient oriented. This means that relationships are a big part of marketing. In fact, it involves all the activities designed to initiate and facilitate building relationships. Any time you are trying to persuade someone to do something you are marketing...whether it is to consider coming to your practice, make the decision to have the recommended treatment completed, keep an appointment, be on time for an appointment, refer another patient, or stay with your practice.

The marketing strategy determines how your practice will fit into the marketplace. You must know the kind of dentistry you want to do and then determine the best way to price, promote and distribute your services. The marketing concept is the philosophy of managing the controllable factors that are at your disposal: product, price, promotion and distribution. When we speak of marketing, it is these four factors with which we are concerned.

Product is the goods or services you have to offer...that means your dentistry and the services you wrap around the actual clinical procedures to complete the total picture. Several questions need to be asked here. How will you package what you have to offer? What range of dental services will you make available? What other services will you offer?

Price is determined by a number of factors. You must consider your quality, the time it takes for you to do a particular procedure, your overhead, as well as what is appropriate in your marketplace for similar services. Too often we pull these numbers out of the air, or allow ourselves to be dicated to by an insurance carrier, or perhaps by comparing our fee schedule with another dentist down the street. Consideration needs to be given here to the factors mentioned in order to price your services fairly, yet profitably.

Distribution refers to the accessibility of your services in relation to your patients. It answers the question, where can I get the service and when is it available. Obviously, your patients must be able to access your dental services from both a time and location perspective.

Promotion refers to a variety of variables involving educating, informing and gaining the agreement of your patients to purchase your services...to have the diagnosed treatment completed. Some of the more typical aspects of promotion involve advertising, publicity, and selling. We'll see how the dental team members are involved in each.

Each of these four factors in the marketing mix should contribute to meeting your practice objectives and at the same time maximize profits.

In order to market your dental practice effectively, your marketing strategy should be well-defined with quantified objectives to measure its success. This means you must know your product. What kinds of dental services do you offer? Do you specialize in any particular area of dentistry? Are you located in a market that can support that specialization? In our competitive environment we must decide how to position ourselves (our practices) in the market. Your services may be wonderful, but the lack of proper marketing (and this does include selling) can doom it to mediocrity...or even failure. It is well worth the time and investment needed to gain the skills and understanding necessary in order to develop a reliable marketing strategy.

The Dental Niche Market

A niche, or target market, is the segment of the market you feel you can serve most effectively. Obviously a practice cannot meet the needs or satisfy all the people all of the time. Further, it is difficult to market by the shotgun approach, hoping to capture the interest of many by being all things to all people. This comes across as vague. Therefore, target marketing comes into play.

Consumers today want to know and feel that products and services are developed with their particular needs in mind. The same is true in dentistry. In order for a patient to choose your practice, they want to know and feel that the type of dentistry they need is what you do very well. They also want to know and feel they will be treated the way they want to be treated. Therefore, it is important to begin by clearly identifying who you want to attract to your practice.

Focusing on a target market accomplishes four things. (1) It focuses business efforts and causes you to establish realistic objectives. (2) It focuses on specific consumer groups which make marketing less expensive and more effective. (3) It helps your practice develop a market niche and differentiates itself from other practices. And (4) it creates a psychological bond with patients that helps them identify with your practice, feeling it is a practice designed especially for them and meets their needs.

There are a variety of factors to consider when identifying a target market. Some of the most common are: Geography (physical location, where you practice dentistry); demographics (age, income level, ethnic group, etc.); personality (psychological needs and wants of potential patients) and specialty (who uses your services and how will they benefit the patient).

The following six question groups follow closely the factors considered above. It is important that you be able to clearly answer these. Failure to understand clearly any one of these could make success much more difficult.

1.   What is my ideal patient profile? Who do we really want to

attract to this practice?

Perhaps you want to attract those interested in cosmetic services or reconstructive cases. Maybe you like to do dentures or veneers. Perhaps you have a different focus. Maybe you prefer working with children, or young adults...or perhaps you best like working with the older patient. Whatever or whoever it is, know who or what it is you want. Of course you must be able to provide your chosen profile with the answers to their needs, wants and desires.

2. Who are my potential patients?

    Without patients there can be no dentistry. It is important to know who your current patients are, and who your target market is (desired patients).

3. Is your target the same as your current patient base?

    If not, this means a change in the dentistry you want to provide, either in the services or type of patient. If this is the case, you must be aware that this will drive other changes in your practice in order to relate to a different market.

4. Why do your patients choose you? What are the key motives for your patients to purchase your dentistry? What needs do you satisfy and does this motivation vary across time, patient profile and market conditions?

    You need to know what is important to your desired patient population. If you prefer working with the elderly, you must know and understand their greatest concerns. Is it reconstruction, dentures or something else? What is it?

5. What are you selling and can you communicate it effec tively?

This means knowing the advantages and disadvantages, as well as the benefits, of your product and service as it relates to your patients and potential patients. You must also be able to communicate to your desired patient population that you can meet their needs.

6. Who is your competition?

    It is important to develop an objective view of your services as well as the services of other dental practices around you. Patients will position your practice in their minds, as well as other practices. How do they view you in relationship to other dental practices? Why would they choose you over the practice down the street? Do you know why? What are your strengths and weaknesses relative to other practices?

You must know your practice thoroughly in order to take full advantage its' strengths (of both product and service) as well as to prepare for handling objections relating to perceived weaknesses.

There is always an element of guesswork in predicting what will happen in the marketplace, and there are many factors affecting demand that are not controllable. They include environmental factors such as cultural, social and economic environment; existing business conditions; and the political and legal environment. But, if you can answer the basic questions, you are on your way to making your practice one that will succeed.

Many practices marketing specific services today (such as implants, reconstructive dentistry, cosmetic dentistry, sealants...even infection control!), both internally and externally, are receiving positive results.

We had the unique experience of being the first in Oregon to have the KCP 2000, allowing Norm to do a great percentage of fillings with no drill and limited, or no, anesthesia. This gave us the opportunity to obtain media coverage, both on television and in the newspaper, regarding this new piece of equipment that was of great interest to a number of people. We received several new patients as a result of this media coverage.

Niche marketing is important in business today and is becoming more important in dentistry, especially in locations where there are an abundance of dentists for the population numbers. Niche means a specific segment of the market. In niche marketing you let your prospective patient population know you have a practice specifically designed for their needs.

Deliver What You Promise

Whatever your message promises to existing or prospective patients, it must be met to maintain credibility and stabilize your position in their minds. If you say you are on time and patients in your office don't wait, then it must be true when they arrive for their appointment. If you say you have a friendly and caring staff, but when the patient arrives at your office they are greeted only when the front office personnel complete their personal conversations, the message earlier communicated will appear bogus. Make sure that whatever you promise you make good in delivery.

Dentists often talk about themselves in the "we" or "our" format. For example, "Our doctors are available 24 hours a day," or "Our staff is well-trained and up-to-date in all aspects of dentistry," or "We have the latest, state-of-the-art equipment." The emphasis is on the organization, but patients will hear everything and see everything through their filter of WIIFM....what's in it for me. To better communicate with the patient, and communicate in a way that grabs the attention, turn it around to WIIFM. The facts don't change, but the orientation does. Instead, say, *"You can feel secure knowing our doctors are available 24 hours a day which means there will be a doctor available when you need one."* Or, *"You can feel confident with our entire team, knowing that each undergoes continual training to remain up-to-date in all aspects of dentistry to provide you the very best treatment possible."*

Patients may be able to make the translation from a "we" statement to the WIIFM...but why leave it to chance? Patients want to know up front and clearly what the benefits are to them. Focus on the "you" rather than the "I" and you will accomplish this easily.

If you don't deliver on that promise you create the opportunity for angry, unhappy people. We develop certain expectations based on what we hear about a business and we enter that business with those expectations. To the extent they are not met, we will be disappointed, and perhaps even angry. If our expectations are met and we receive *nothing more and nothing less* than we expect, then we fall into the neutral zone. Even this is not safe for our dental practices today. The first time a "neutral zone" patient is coaxed by a patient who is super enthusiastic about another practice, you run the risk of losing that patient. But, when we have certain expectations, and feel it is worthwhile to give that business a try, and then our *expectations are exceeded*...that's when the magic happens. That's when the unsolicited referrals begin to appear.

Unfortunately, however, much money is spent in getting patients in the door, but so little training is done to help the employee know how to treat the patient when he or she calls or walks through the door.

**No matter how great your marketing program,
if you get patients in the door but can't keep them there
you've lost all the way around.**

It is what you have created inside your office that will keep them returning and allow you to draw even more referrals.

The Invisibility Factor

Dentistry can be quite invisible...unless and until you make it visible. No matter how good your work is and how great your staff is, if other people don't hear about you or know about you, new patients will only trickle in. In my years as sales manager for a national insurance firm, I used to tell my agents, "No matter how good you are at sales, and no matter how great you are with people, if no one knows about you, *if you play secret agent*, you'll never be successful." The same goes for our dental practices. People have to know about you and hear about you, and when they do it must be in a way that gets their attention. That's positioning...that's marketing.

Also often invisible to the patient is the benefit of dentistry. Remember, the benefits of dentistry are much more apparent to you than to your patient. While you take great pride in sculpting a restoration, or preparing a crown with excellent margins, to the patient it is "just a filling" or "just a crown." They don't understand (most never have, and most never will) all that is required to achieve the end result, to make the occlusion exactly right, so they *don't feel the filling or the crown*. Amazing isn't it, that you spend so much time working on something hoping that the patient won't even know it's there!

To further complicate the invisibility problem, because not much has been done in the way of marketing (including advertising, sales, etc.), the dental profession has allowed others, by default, to portray an image that is one of pain, of comparing the negative things in life to dentistry. How many times do we hear "I'd rather do......than sit in a dentist's chair," or "It's just like pulling teeth to get......" The images portrayed are not positive. Yet, because of the limited visibility on the positive side, this is the image that has stuck in the "public's" mind and how dentistry has been perceived by so many people.

Consider, too, the terminology that does dentistry a disservice. For example, how many practices refer to a prophylaxis as a "cleaning" or a "recall" appointment. Cleaning has several connotations...usually a chore, not necessarilly fun. Cleaning also suggests that something is dirty...and people don't like to feel dirty. Or in many instances the feeling might simply be, "I clean my teeth every day by brushing, therefore the cleaning appointment isn't urgent and I can put it off." Or what about the word "recall." What do people outside the dental profession think of when they hear "recall?" Of course, something is defective. They recall cars and trucks; they recall ceiling fans and numerous other products. Why would anyone get excited about a "recall" appointment? Habit has gotten us into this situation...and changing the habit will get us out. Our words paint a picture and when it isn't a compelling, emotional picture, the need or treatment becomes nonessential in the patient's mind. The result is people putting off their appointments or cancelling at the last minute when something more interesting or perceived as more important comes up.

Another aspect of terminology surfaces when you consider *how* you target the market you are after. For example...perhaps you have a practice geared toward the geriatric patient. You might be tempted to use that term in written materials, brochures or advertising of any other kind. You understand it, your colleagues understand it, and your patients or prospective patients will probably understand it...but they most likely won't like it! Geriatric speaks of "old." And regardless of age, many people don't feel comfortable or want to be reminded of age. Therefore, talk about what *benefits* you have to offer those particular patients. Position yourself positively with a different image. Talk about implants, helping people feel comfortable and enjoy their leisure time. Talk about helping them be able to once again eat foods they've been unable to touch. Let them know you are accessible when they need you and that you have "years of experience." Communicate that you have several financial options available for their dentistry.

Norm had the experience of one female patient showing up in the office following extensive reconstructive work...with two huge T-bone steaks and a wonderful card. On the inside of the card she wrote, "Roses are red, violets are blue, other people eat steak, now I can too!"

She was very grateful for what Norm gave her back the ability to do. She was an older woman, yes. But she didn't consider herself old. She was an active, vivacious, outgoing woman full of life. And she received, through dentistry and Norm's capabilities, her dream come true.

Never once did the practice team or Norm or any of the practice marketing materials speak to geriatric dentistry. Instead, the emphasis was on what we could provide in the way of benefits. When this women understood that there could be a better way, she was ready and willing...and was one enthusiastic lady following the treatment.

Another perception people in this country have is that tooth loss goes right along with the aging process. They still haven't made the connection that they lose their teeth because the teeth and gums are not properly cared for. Therefore, many erroneously believe (and approximately half the American public does not see a dentist), whether or not they go to the dentist won't have any affect on how long they will keep their teeth. Yet, marketing research definitely shows that most people want to keep their teeth. In fact, the thought of dentures or "false teeth" is actually repulsive to many. So, whose job is it? It is our job, every person in the dental profession, to make the connection. We must educate our patients. We must make our mark and we must communicate in order to do so.

Understand that even the most voraciously vocal dentist *against* advertising markets! You can't help it. You and your staff market 100% of the time you are in the practice, every single day. And outside the practice. Every member of your staff is an ambassador for the practice. What do your materials look like? Your cards, letterhead, brochures and every other piece of written material that goes out of your office. Does it create the image you want it to create? Is it dog-eared, out of date, full of typographical errors? How does your office look? When patients enter through the front door, does it invite them inside, or does it portray a cold, distant feeling? Is it clean, or disorderly? What image does your physical space create? And what about the appearance of your team members? Are they well-groomed, neat, pleasant looking? Or do they look like they jumped out of the bed at the last minute and raced to the office, without much attention to the image they are projecting? And what about their faces, body language, tone of voice? What kind of image is being created? How is the telephone answered? How are you being positioned in the minds of your patients and potential patients? And has it been by choice...or by default? Are your patients put off by your fees simply because they don't perceive any difference between your practice and the one down the street? Many dentists still haven't addressed the image factor of their practice, but few of us today have the luxury to sit by without caring, at least if we want to have a successful, profitable practice. Dentists who pay no attention to their image, to how they are being perceived, to their positioning, are apt to lose patients to low-fee providers next door.

> You are continually marketing your practice
> each and every day, consciously or unconsciously,
> through your actions, appearance, behavior, and surroundings.

Does the patient in your chair feel that he or she is the most important patient you have that day? Do your patients feel this is the very best practice they could possibly select? And are you giving them reasons to feel this way? Look at your practice and yourself the way a patient does. What are you communicating by your conversation, your appearance, your body language? And look at each employee with this perspective. It will make a difference!

Perhaps it is time to walk in the front door and enter as though you are a patient, when the staff at the front desk is unaware. Or maybe it is time to call in to see how the phone is answered, or have a friend call and see how they are treated. Know what it feels like to be a patient in your practice, or a potential patient calling for the first time. Know how you are being positioned...quietly, invisibly, every moment of every day.

The bottom line to the marketing issue is that in order for you to stand out to your patients, to draw referrals and other new sources of patients, you want your practice to have personality...a defined image. You want it to be visible, not invisible. This is making your mark. This is increasing your visibility. When you have done this succesfully, people will have something to refer to. Think about it for a moment. If all that stands out in your patient's mind is that he hasn't had any problem with you or your staff, if he thinks you're a nice person but can't put into words what makes you different, then why would he even bring up your name to someone who might otherwise be a referral?

Methods of Marketing: Internal and External, Passive and Active

Before we consider a number of methods to market your practice, remember once again that it is not worth investing in external forms of marketing until your internal marketing is in place and in good shape. The following gives several suggestions for marketing. It is quite obvious that no one practice will employ every one of these marketing methods. Instead, consider your own practice, your market, your staff and how you operate. Then choose a limited number from among these, or perhaps others that you have identified, and develop a plan for following through.

We'll begin with the active forms of marketing. These are the methods that require you to take the first step.

Internally generated referrals. Every patient gained from an external source, or any other source, should be multiplied through referrals. If not, then you are wasting your dollars on any form of external marketing. Referrals are the most effective, least costly method of marketing and bringing new patients into your practice. Because it is, I include it as one of the nine steps in the selling process. We'll devote all of chapter 30 to referrals.

Most practices generate much less than one referral per patient per year, yet it is a well known and accepted fact that we each have a circle of influence that extends to approximately 250 people. Each and every person has this circle of influence. Therefore, we have a long way to go!

Why aren't referrals happening? The reason is, I believe, that we haven't built our practices in such a way that people *can't help but talk about them.* When we do, we will see the referrals coming in the door on a regular basis. Once we have that dynamic, enthusiastic, dramatically different practice, all we'll need to do to gain a regular flow of referrals is to let our patients know we would appreciate their referrals. In order to get to this point, however, you must do what you do so well that people can't help but talk about you. And this, of course, means much more than the technical skills. In fact, the technical skills are the one thing most patients have no clue about! It's the customer service or patient relations aspect we'll cover in chapters 35 through 37 that will make a tremendous difference. But just for now, remember that you must be so good they can't help but talk about you.

Norm and I knew what we wanted to build with our practice. And we knew we could not build it ourselves; it would take our efforts, as well as those of every employee in our practice. Therefore, we first concentrated on finding employees who were right for our practice. Our practice...not some other practice. Our staff is handpicked very carefully. We go through a relatively long interview process, as discussed in Part Two, and use the time as a "courtship period" to see if it will be a good "marriage."

We both realize that with the right employees for our practice, we will be happy, they will be happy, the patients will be happy and the practice can continually grow and flourish. That means we must share similar values, philosophy and attitudes toward not only dentistry, but about patient care and a general philosophy toward life. We find that by selecting carefully we can literally build a practice "family." It isn't an easy task, but the efforts, time and dollars invested are well worth it.

As a team, we all agreed on what we wanted to give to our patients. And what we came up with was, "An Exceptional Dental Experience." The entire team was so committed to making this a constant in the practice, and so confident that we could measure up every time, that we began utilizing this phrase on all the practice written materials. This tells our patients, existing and potential, what they can expect. As new or existing patients come into our practice, our dental team makes sure they are not disappointed.

In the earlier chapters on mission and vision, it was pointed out that where the team has a passion for a common vision, any dream can come true. When the team members have a passion for the vision it automatically creates enthusiasm. A vision with passion finds a way around, over or through obstacles. It makes the impossible possible. And that's what has happened with our *"An Exceptional Dental Experience."*

Our patients know the difference. They feel it when they call on the phone. They feel it when they walk in the door. They experience it every minute they are in the practice...whether they are with the administrative coordinator, clinical chairside assistant, hygienist or dentist.

It is not uncommon for us to receive notes or letters of thanks, directed to the entire team or to a particular employee or to Norm. The bottom line is that patients get more than they expect, and they like it! As a result, they refer new patients to us continually.

Referrals generated by your staff from patients is the least costly, most effective form of marketing you can do.

Go through existing charts for incomplete treatment. Make this a part of every morning huddle. Check for treatment diagnosed but not completed on every patient coming in that day. Then, be sure to discuss it with the patient and encourage them to schedule the needed treatment. If you have a cancellation during the day, and it creates additional time for one of those patients with needed treatment, take the extra time (with the patients okay, of course) to do it right then. You'll want to make sure, of course, that the patient's financial account is current before additional fees are incurred.

Beyond the morning huddle, map out a plan to go through your entire active patient files and check for incomplete treatment. Then contact these patients to let them know of your concern for them and their dental health, and work to get them scheduled. Most dental practices that have been around a few years have a wealth of inventory in their existing charts. Take time to identify the literally thousands and hundreds of thousands of dollars of diagnosed but uncompleted treatment in the charts. Realize that the longer the treatment is put off, the bigger the problem that may be created for the patient.

Patient newsletters. Newsletters keep your practice in the forefront of your patients' minds. Many people use them with great results. The informational nature in a newsletter does not suggest advertising. It is educational, telling what is new and noteworthy in dentistry. This serves to inform and remind your patients of the services you perform. If you choose not to do a newsletter on a regular basis throughout the year, perhaps you might choose to do one only once or twice a year at a specific time such as the Thanksgiving-Christmas holiday time or New Year's, or even Easter or Spring or whatever other time of the year you want to tie your message into. Obviously, every article should emphasize quality dentistry and professional caring.

Another idea is to send a newsletter to someone other than your patients. For example, why not send a newsletter to physicians on the latest research finding concerning matters about which they are being questioned by their patients, such as occlusal sealants, supplemental fluoride, nursing bottle syndrome, mouth guards for contact sports, etc. Explain new procedures and give updates on equipment or infection control measures. And, of course, enclose several business cards.

A variation of the newsletter is a letter sent to patients periodically over the course of a year, updating them on advances in periodontics, cosmetics, equipment or any other appropriate topic.

Perhaps you might want to use a "have a great summer" or "all the best in the new year" type letter just to stay in touch...and to let your patients know that you would consider it a privilege to serve anyone they refer.

Practice brochures. Brochures are important, but keep them clean and simple. If they become too long and windy they may not get read. Patients don't have the time, patience, and many times the interest, to read something that is long and involved. If you have a brochure, ask your patients if they have read it. It will give you some good clues. And what about the tone in which it is written? Does it sound like it is a set of policies that are cold and extremely rigid, or does the brochure communicate warmth and welcoming?

A brochure reduces the need for repetitive explanation of routine information, saving time and allowing for greater office efficiency. A brochure should orient a new patient to the practice and provide relevant information for current patients. It also helps prevent misunderstandings and establishes certain expectations. Once again, remember to meet or exceed the patients' expectations you have created to keep them happy and coming back.

If you choose to have a brochure produced, be sure to get help writing the copy so it achieves your purpose and informs in a way that persuades the patient your practice is the place to be.

Reactivating old patients. Many patients are lost in the files. Perhaps they were never followed up because of a misunderstanding or unpleasant experience that occurred the last time they were in and the staff would just as soon forget about the situation. Perhaps it is simply because there has been no system to keep them from falling through the cracks. Nevertheless, there could be a goldmine in your files from just such patients.

When the decision is made to recontact these patients hoping to reactivate them, a mistake is often made. Sometimes this is considered a "drudgery job" and is given to some staff member as an "add on project." In other words, calling these patients is given to the part-time high school assistant, or to the roving chairside assistant who has extra time. But think about it. Reactivating these people is an important responsibility and it calls for *the very best communicator* you have to get the job done, and done effectively. This person should be someone who has great communication skills, dental experience, and a warm, friendly personality that comes across on the phone. If you have a larger practice with more team members, and you have more than one who fits into this category, you can reactivate with a team approach.

Prior to beginning reactivation, be sure to have a heart-to-heart discussion about letting go of the negative attitudes surrounding reactivation. Then, as the process is begun, it might be a good idea to have a check-in periodically to see what obstacles the individual doing the work might be running up against. It is imperative that the chart always be in front of the caller when talking with the patient. It is a good idea, not only for your documentation, but for the caller's own feedback, to have some kind of tracking form. This can be very simple. Make a page with column headings of patient, treatment needed, last hygiene appointment and when next due, date appointment scheduled, and comments.

Include in the comments if the patient has moved, gone to another dentist, etc. Find out why they are leaving or have left.

Mrs. Jones, I'm very sorry to hear you feel our fees are too high. Doctor is concerned about providing his patients with the very best quality of care, and our entire team is totally committed to making each of your visits to our office a pleasant experience.

May I ask you, are you receiving (and mention a service/benefit you provide....such as oral cancer screening, etc.) at each appointment where you are now going?

We want you to know that if you should ever like to return to our practice we would consider it a privilege to serve you again.

As the reactivation call is made, be sure the individual making the calls comes across as warm, friendly and concerned.

I was reviewing the records and I notice that you haven't been in for quite some time. We've missed you, and Doctor is concerned about (the particular dental concern).

This takes some time, but often this is a great way to increase your production and move your practice forward again.

Networking. Networking with potential referral sources is another form of marketing. This could be with any number of individuals such as plastic surgeons, pediatricians, pharmacists, school nurses, etc. People associated with healthcare in some form are great networking sources. Networking means being in the appropriate places to be in contact with these people, become known, and eventually gaining the respect and hopefully referrals. These contacts may be made individually over breakfast or lunch, or a quick "coffee" meeting to introduce yourself and discuss the possibility of how you can help each other. Once you identify potential patients or sources of referrals through your networking, it is important that you follow-up the initial contact.

Perhaps you work in a building that houses many healthcare professionals. Are these individuals you would like to associate with and perhaps cooperatively market by distributing each other's brochures in your offices?

Be creative here, there are many ways of getting the word out about your practice. Some of these methods will no doubt seem very uncomfortable when you first consider them. Just remember, that's most likely because it isn't something you have previously done. We can never learn to do anything well unless we are willing to step out of our comfort zone and do what is uncomfortable, and do it enough times until we begin doing it well...and then it will become comfortable!

Many business people join organizations of all types to network. Whether it be a Rotary, Kiwanis, Chamber of Commerce, Toastmasters, a church group, a philanthropic organization, or any other type, it is important that you have a desire to truly help and do your part in the organization. If you join solely for the purpose of gaining new patients, it will come across that way and the first impression will be one you'd rather not make!

Networking takes time and effort that is required to attend meetings, be involved on committees, etc.

Direct mail. Quality and perceived sincerity of the message have great impact when using direct mail. One key to a successful direct mail marketing program is repetition. It is important that the individual to whom the direct mail is being sent see your name at least three times in order for it to become "familiar."

Direct mail can be a specific letter or brochure targeting a specific market or audience at a particular time of the year (holidays, summer, National Dental Health Week, etc). It can be an announcement of the opening of your new office or location, or an announcement of new equipment, or whatever you feel is appropriate to let your existing and/or prospective patients know about you and your practice. It might even be a special message or announcement you make via a statement stuffer.

Direct mail allows you the opportunity to target particular groups. You may want to send direct mail with one message to elderly people, and a different message to those you feel would be interested in cosmetic dentistry. Direct mail needs to be developed properly in order to get your greatest return. Make sure you get some help with this if you are unfamiliar with direct mail. The message must be clear and delivered with impact. Further, if you are going to purchase lists for use with your direct mail, make sure you have an appropriate list! There are a number of consultants or direct mail houses who can help you develop your direct mail program.

As soon as we moved to our new location we contacted, by letter, every business on the hill where the practice was located, which involves around 1,000 employees. It wasn't a quick fix, but people did begin calling the practice as a perceived need arose. We now have a substantial number of local employees in the practice, and they are referring not only fellow employees, but other people they know.

If you choose to be involved in a direct mail campaign, make sure the entire staff is involved so when inquiries are received, whether over the phone or in person, they will be prepared to handle them. Remember: repeat your direct mail campaign in cycles. A single mailer is not sufficient to yield the greatest results. Be specific. Distinguish yourself from other dental practices. Focus on the benefits that fit your target market's needs.

Although some people have chosen direct mail as a marketing method, and have achieved varying levels of success, be aware that direct mail is a time, labor, and dollar intensive method of marketing.

Special occasion letters or direct mail. There are several occasions throughout the year where direct mail would be appropriate. Some are with current patients, and others are for prospective patients. For example, you could send a letter a few months before the end of the year to patients with dental insurance as a reminder that the end of the year is rapidly approaching and now is the time to schedule any unscheduled treatment if they want to use the remaining insurance benefits...a "use it or lose it" approach.

Another example involves the many massive layoffs that continue to occur within companies throughout the nation. If you hear of such an action being taken in the next month or two or three in your area, why not contact any patients you may have who work for that company and remind them to get in while their insurance benefits are still in effect. You can ask them for referrals to other individuals in the company as well. Many computer programs allow you to pull all the patients who work with a particular company so you have a list from which to work.

Along the same line, contact patients with dental insurance who did not complete treatment during the past year because they ran out of insurance benefits. Remind them that a new year has begun and insurance benefits for the year begin anew. (Obviously these patients haven't yet learned that dental needs aren't based on what benefit the insurance company will pay, or fall into neatly divided financial categories from year to year! These patients need further dental education.)

Informational presentations. Here you could identify a certain segment of your patient population whom you feel would be interested in a particular service, and then invite them in for a presentation in a small group format on that service. You could take this further and do a direct mail piece to a targeted market and invite those individuals in for a similar type presentation.

Other presentations might include making yourself available to local organizations (most are always looking for speakers) to present a program on a dental subject of interest to their members, such as implants, cosmetic dentistry, bleaching, gum disease, etc. Or perhaps you could visit the local schools in your area to do a dental health presentation.

Finally, there are many sources from which you can develop your list for prospective patients: mailing houses, telephone company, and utility companies to name a few.

After moving to our new practice location, and wanting to attract individuals from the immediate area, we purchased the "new mover list" from the telephone company. We were able to select only those people who lived in single family dwellings and who own (or were purchasing) their homes in the four zip code areas directly surrounding our practice. These people were sent a letter introducing and welcoming them to our practice.

Direct contact or cold calls. Direct contact means approaching businesses, offices and shops to let them know of your services. The most likely would be those in close geographic proximity to your practice. Again, you must be able to present yourself and your practice in such a way that is different, that would give them a reason to consider choosing your practice over another down the street.

One example of a direct contact would be to contact the person responsible for human resources in a large corporation or business within a reasonable distance from your practice. Find out who the person is, what insurance program they have (to determine if it is a dental maintenance organization or capitation plan) and then invite them to lunch to introduce yourself and your practice. Perhaps you might want to take one of your employees along. Here's an example of how this can work.

We heard that a nearby hospital was changing dental insurance plans, which opened the doors for their employees to choose other providers. Our hygienist knew the human resource person and scheduled a luncheon appointment for the two of them and Norm to get together. After lunch they came back to the office for a tour. The result? The human resource manager is a now a patient, as well as her husband, and we have received several referrals from both.

Show and tell. Put together a *before and after* notebook showing patients the dental services available. Likewise, compile a list of all the topics you wish to educate your patients about, write text about each area and put it together with pictures to substantiate and illustrate the treatment where possible. This is a great educational tool, as well as a marketing and selling tool. Consider also putting together a behind-the-scenes section on infection control in your practice. Have photos showing exactly how you sterilize instruments, disinfect operatories, plastic wrap x-ray controls, and whatever else you want to show your patients.

In another section, or distributed throughout the book in an appropriate area, include testimonials from patients. These could be about your professionalism, courtesy, meeting their needs, personal caring by you and your staff, or anything else you are commended for. Make sure the person giving the testimonial knows how and where it will be used, and get their approval in writing. State the testimonial correctly and have the patient review it for accuracy. Don't use testimonials that guarantee or suggest clinical outcome, but do include those that relate to their feelings of satisfaction for the work performed and those pertaining to the personal characteristics of your staff and your overall practice.

Television and radio. This is more expensive advertising, and is usually not practical for the smaller office. If you are part of a larger clinic, or have several locations in the area and wish to have your message communicated to the entire community, this form of advertising might be appropriate.

Print media. Newspaper advertising may or may not be appropriate in your locale. Some areas allow targeting by placing an ad in a special section that is distributed only to a particular area. If you live in a smaller community where the whole town is in reasonable proximity to your office, the newspaper might be a great way to let people know of your presence.

Shared marketing. If you have other healthcare practitioners with whom you feel comfortable associating, you might consider developing a shared marketing effort where together you promote your practices, and thereby reduce the cost to each of you as you reach the target audience. This cooperative approach can work with a number of marketing approaches. A combined brochure that covers each practitioner can be distributed from each practice allowing visibility among a greater number of patients.

Sharing a newsletter with tips from each speciality is also a possibility. No one practice has to come up with all the information so it is less time consuming, as well as sharing the costs of printing and distribution if you choose to do a direct type mailing effort.

If the shared marketing approach appeals to you, go through the list of marketing ideas and determine which methods would work for your shared marketing program. Brainstorm with your chosen affiliated practitioners and you'll probably come up with a number of others.

Business cards. Make your business card work for you. Carry it with you wherever you go. Have cards made for your staff. Make sure no appropriate opportunity passes by without distributing your cards. Business cards can be very useful, and they can be a silent marketer for your practice.

The list goes on. There are numerous other marketing ideas, limited only by your creativity. Advertising in the yellow pages or other area directories; referral signs in your office letting patients know you appreciate their referrals; sending birthday cards; calling back patients who no show for their appointment; video presentations for patient education; patient referral programs (there are several around the country); and flowers for patients as they come in for appointments (done every day or just for special holiday occasions) are just a few. Also consider an appreciation gift for those who refer to you continually, as well as a thank you card for every person who refers someone to your practice. Remember, behavior that is rewarded gets repeated!

You Make the Choice

Patients expectations are changing, and with them the ground rules for success. The result is that many of the marketing ideas of days gone by are yielding only minimal results today. Yellow pages advertising, mass mailings and other forms of self-promotion don't provide the return they once did. Surveys indicate that except for low price (fee) advertising, the returns are extremely low in the new patients they generate, and in the retention of those patients. Marquette University School of Dentistry reports that only six percent of patients use the Yellow Pages. The ADA/Gallup poll of early 1992 indicates five percent. If 95% of your patients are referred, is it worth the time, effort and dollars it costs to advertise to attract the other five or six percent? Only you can make your decision.

Marketing the Practice in Tough Times

When the economy is at a low and times seem tough, first remember that much of it is a matter of attitude. If any one of your patients went to a physician and was told he or she needed immediate surgery, would they be likely to tell the physician that "times are tough and I really need to hold off on this?" Probably not. It would most likely be a priority and the patient would find a way to have the surgery completed.

When times are tough, redefine the value of your services for your patients in your practice or in your market area. Boost the level of value the patient expects and how the dentistry is delivered by creating a new expectation in their mind. Today's consumers have an expanded concept of value that includes convenience of purchase, after the sale service, dependability, and "extra mile service." Become champions of excellence. Deliver superior customer service to your patients operationally (meaning a specific strategic approach to providing dental services), patient relations (continually make sure you relate the need for the service to the patients interests...we'll discuss this in upcoming chapters), talk about lifetime value and how it is achieved, and provide state-of-the art dental products and services.

During tough times it may appear that patients don't have the money to pay for *needed* services. But they will pay for what they *want*. (In the several chapters on sales we'll dicuss how to find their hot buttons and relate their needs to what they want.) The elective type procedures may seem to be the least likely desired services in a down economy. Actually, they can be some of the best!

Esthetic dentistry provides an example. Bonding, bleaching, crown and bridge and porcelain-laminate veneers may provide the boost that people want. In a down time people will actually look for things to give them a boost mentally and emotionally, and improving their appearance fits into this category. Focus on the patient's main goals. If the patient wants an enhanced smile, concentrate on what the final result will be. Use models, before and after photos, pictures and drawings to demonstrate the result.

When times are tough it is not time to pull back your marketing efforts, but a time to be more proactive. Here are some factors to consider:

Be positive. Your attitude becomes a self-fulfilling prophecy. Remember the speed of the leader is the speed of the pack.

Do not lower your fees. Low fees do not attract most patients. The perception of your quality may drop if you lower your fees. It is also necessary that you maintain your profit level to keep pace with any potential rise in costs from suppliers to you.

Work on interpersonal skills. Communicatoin is incredibly important. Every person in the practice needs to work on this area. A receptionist with fine people skills can help you close sales, as can the assistant and hygienist. Every patient must be celebrated and treatment maximized.

Have options for payment. This doesn't mean you have to finance the patients treatment in-house, but you do need to provide optional methods for your patients such as healthcare credit cards and the more traditional credit cards.

Increase your selling time by 200-300 percent. Have every staff person take a more active role here. Time spent in the hygienist's chair should be spent on patient education, not idle chatter. The receptionist can talk with the patient about their concerns, desires, etc. and pass that on to you. The assistant can be right there to back up your recommendation with her agreement.

Increase your hygiene production. Eighty-five to ninety-five percent of all adults suffer from varying degrees of periodontal disease, according to some studies. Make sure you are offering patient education and taking care of your patients periodontically.

Monitor your new patient statistics. Are you doing complete new patient exams? Are you diagnosing and recommending comprehensive treatment that is truly needed? And what about your treatment plan acceptance percentage? Perhaps it is time to work on some of the selling skills.

Increase the TLC factor. Nurture your patients. Call in the entire staff to see the great bridge you just placed or to see how beautifully the crown matches the rest of the teeth. Do whatever you can to make the patient feel good about the treatment they have chosen. Help them feel good about investing in their treatment. Follow up appropriate procedures with calls after treatment to see how the patient is doing, hand write a note to thank the referrers of patients, and take before and after photos for your patients.

Put your computer to work. Maximize your hygiene appointments and make sure you follow up on any incomplete treatment plans.

Market, market, market!

These are all areas that should be a normal part of your everyday practice. But if they are not, and you are having trouble with your results, pay some attention to each. How your practice is affected by a recession or a down economy depends more on how you choose to think and respond than on the economy itself.

Summary

Abraham Maslow once said, "Always deal with reality, not with what you think should be true, not what you wish were true, not what was true, but what is true." If what you are doing isn't working, or isn't getting you the results you want, do something different! It may be stressful considering philosophies different from what you are used to considering, but by increasing your level of tolerance for that which is "different," you may also increase the productivity of your practice. Consider all the different methods of marketing and select those that mesh with your personality, service mix, and professional goals and objectives.

A balanced business in these critical areas that comprise the marketing mix doesn't just happen. And profits don't just happen. It takes careful, well thought out planning to get the results you want, to build the practice of your dreams. Continuing evaluation is necessary in order to adapt to or produce new products or services to meet new and changing demands, increased competition, and new technology. Every practice owner should continue analysis and evaluation on a regular basis as the practice grows and changes, and as the market changes. What worked yesterday may not (and in our changing world probably will not) be the formula for tomorrow. Be responsive to those areas which impact your particular patient base. Monitor and respond as accurately as possible to the times. And you'll then have many of the necessary ingredients to "keep on succeeding."

Many practices have great marketing programs and generate a healthy new patient flow as a result. There are, however, numerous practices where not enough attention is given to retaining those patients once they have entered the practice, and that's still marketing. It's expensive to bring a new patient into the practice, and retention is important in making the initial investment pay dividends. Just as we'll see in the next several chapters, closing begins at the beginning, and retention of your patients begins with the first impression the patient has of your practice, whether it is in person, on the telephone, in writing, or from an oral introduction by another person or patient.

Perhaps the most important point to be made about marketing has to do with your attitude and the attitude of your team. All the marketing tools in the world won't help, not for very long, if the attitude isn't right.

> We attract what we focus on;
> energy flows to where the concentration goes.

If you're not getting the new patient flow you really want; if you're not getting the treatment acceptance you desire; if you find patients coming in only once or twice and not returning, the place to begin...FIRST...is within. What are your attitudes about what you do? What are the attitudes of your staff? Who are you attracting to your practice? What kinds of problems, difficulties or obstacles are you attracting to you? What attitudes do you have about what and who you believe you will attract?

Marketing is important. And you do it every day. You, every associate dentist in your practice, every employee, and every spouse is an ambassador for your practice. What signals are they sending? What message are they sending? Make sure it is the one you want to project.

Chapter 23

INTRODUCTION TO THE PRINCIPLED SELLING PROCESS

Albert Schweitzer, speaking to a group of college students said, "I do not know what your destiny will be, but I do know this: that the only ones of you who will be happy are those who have sought and found out how to serve."

Selling is not about hard sell or soft sell...it is about serving, educating, communicating and building relationships. Many healthcare professionals don't like the word sell, but like it or not we are all salespeople. Every time you present a treatment plan or discuss treatment in any way, you are selling. You and your staff are selling when you communicate to your patients the importance of their next visit, whether it be for restorative work or hygiene. Your receptionist sells every time she answers the phone or makes an outgoing call. Your financial person is selling every time she discusses payment options with your patients. Everyone is selling! And if you're not paying attention to how it is being done, you may be experiencing low new patient flow, rejected treatment plans, cancellations, failed appointments, collection problems...and probably low morale.

Let's clarify exactly what we mean by sales.

A sale is a value judgment arrived at in the
mind of a person (a prospective or current patient) with
the ability to buy.

Nothing more, nothing less. It is a *value judgment.* In other words, when I, as the patient or prospective patient, come to believe that what is being presented for sale is something I need or want, and I believe that the value is equal to or greater than the price I will have to pay for it, then I will most likely buy. I have arrived at a value judgment in my mind that says it's a good trade. And that's exactly what you do in dentistry. You help people arrive at the value judgment that the treatment plan you are presenting is what is needed, wanted, and worth the trade of dollars for service.

Every person alive is a salesperson. We must sell in order to survive and live in this world. We sell all day, every day...to staff, superiors, spouses, children...you name it. We are selling many things although we don't recognize it as selling...our appearance and dress, our manners, our communication, our optimism, and our mental attitude towards everything. We sell our thoughts, our experiences, our skills and abilities, and all that we are.

Kiwi International Airlines has a philosophy that everyone sells. They have a job description and the responsibilities that go with every posi-tion, including their sales responsibilities. Pilots, mechanics, flight attendants, reservation agents, corporate executives...everyone...must sell. Selling is considered a point of honor at Kiwi.

There is nothing wrong with selling. In fact, it is a very noble calling. Nothing would ever happen in this world, personally or professionally, if there was no selling. Ministers sell, doctors sell, attorneys sell, accountants sell, and your children sell! Sometimes we confuse selling and financial success with something negative. The only time we have to apologize for our success is when our success is a failure. Orison Swett Marden in 1906 said, "When is success a failure? When you go on the principle of getting all you can and giving as little as possible in return."

Many dentists spend a great amount of time and dollars taking continuing education courses. They perfect, upgrade, or learn new clinical skills, only to discover back at the office that they don't feel confident, and are therefore uncomfortable, in presenting major treatment plans and gaining patient acceptance. Not having the selling skills results in not being able to do the kind of dentistry you would like to and are qualified to do. And that creates stress, frustration, and even depression.

> Successful people are motivated by pleasing *results*.
> Those who have settled for mediocrity or failure
> are motivated by pleasing *methods*.

The pleasing methods are doing what is quick, easy and fun, or at least known. Pleasing results are practicing the kind of dentistry you choose...and getting the desired results. But to get the pleasing results means investing whatever it takes to make it happen. It involves taking the time to learn and practice sales skills. It isn't necessarily quick or easy, and certainly it is not known to most dentists today. And it probably won't be fun until you begin doing it, practicing it, and begin to have some successes. Then it will be great fun!

In my business it would be nice if I all I had to do was show up and speak, train, or consult, but I have to get the lead or respond to a referral, follow up on it, qualify it, match my service to the needs and then close the sale. That's what any business is about, including dentistry.

Sales and marketing are no longer an option in dentistry, but a necessity. What has passed for sales in the past has been order taking: allowing the patients to tell you what they want of your diagnosed treatment, and accepting their order. In order to do what is *best* for our patients, however, most often we must sell.

Before we get into the actual sales process, there are a number of factors to be aware of that will directly affect the outcome of the selling process.

Selling is educating. We must educate our patients. Our society has changed and we are in a period of renewal, growth and retraining. People today are more knowledgeable and sophisticated than in previous generations. Our patients are more educated about choices because of the information available to them via television, radio, print media, telephone solicitation, direct mail, educational programs on cable, and other sources of exposure. It doesn't necessarily mean they understand, but they are no longer willing to accept recommended treatment just because their doctor says it is necessary. They want to understand consequences. They want choices and options. They want to feel they are in control. And the dental practice of the 21st century must respond by focusing on the benefits to the patients. Although we have always sold in dentistry, traditional selling was accomplished by the dentist simply telling the patient what he or she needed. No longer can we *tell*; we must *sell.*

Selling isn't manipulation. The purpose of selling is to create value for the patient. The selling process revolves around partnering with your patient to create value together.

Creating values requires that we raise our standards about the contributions we make, how we interact with our patients, our own character and integrity, and the value we place on the patient-doctor-staff relationship. The reality is such that when a patient is in partnership with you they are making themselves vulnerable. They are opening to you with their life and entrusting you with information about themselves. Unless they trust you and feel you will make recommendations based on their best interests, unless you treat them with total integrity, you'll never be in partnership. You'll be on the outside trying to pull them in.

We need to remember the root meaning of the word doctor....*to teach.* Selling is about educating and teaching.

A colleague of mine, Fred M., shared this most revealing story with me. Fred grew up in a family that was very concerned about cleanliness. Yet, in all his years of visiting his dentist, no one ever educated him on brushing and flossing. Oh yes, Fred brushed, but not understanding how to brush, and never knowing about flossing, his homecare obviously suffered. The result? He has very few natural teeth left.

As an adult at 65, Fred went to a new dentist. This dentist had a totally different approach. One of the first things the new dentist said to him was this, "Fred, those few remaining teeth are important. And I'm going to help you and show you how you can save them."

Fred says, "I felt so guilty. It was as though I was dirty. I didn't know why I was losing my teeth. I had no idea that I wasn't doing what was necessary to keep my teeth. Now that my new dentist has not only explained to me how to take care of my remaining teeth, but has shown me how to brush and floss...now I actually get commended for the care I am giving to the natural teeth I have left."

We do have an obligation. It is a wonderful privilege to have our patients entrust to us their dental care. And with that privilege comes a responsibility. We must educate our patients. That doesn't mean we go through a one-time homecare program. It is an ongoing process. We should develop a continuing education philosophy and every time the patient is in our office that education should continue.

We must be patient oriented. Selling requires a good understanding of people or interpersonal skills. In our attempts to restore a patient to good oral health, we must not overlook the compassion and understanding that is so necessary to building trust and good relationships. The doctor of old was known for his "bedside manner." Translated, that means interpersonal or people skills. Perhaps they could offer nothing more than compassion, hope, and a genuine sense of caring. In fact, the old fashioned rural "Doc" was assumed to be a friend in whom one could place ultimate trust, as well as feel confident of the Doc's knowledge. The general public has the image that in today's modern practice the "Doc" has all but disappeared.

Although technical knowledge has increased tremendously and diagnostic techniques have changed dramatically, many feel that we've lost something the "Doc" of old gave to us...careful listening and empathic response. A survey today might well identify that patients have no problem with the competence and expertise of their physician or dentist, but they may indicate a dissatisfaction with the human element. And what's more, they don't just expect it from the doctor, but from the entire team. Patients today want a chance to talk, to be listened to, to be educated, to be cared about...and to feel safe to ask a question without fear that you or a team member will think it is "dumb or stupid." When this doesn't happen, they feel a missing link; expectations are higher than reality, and that's where the dissatisfaction begins.

When we make our patients the central focus of our concern when we are with them, when they feel like they are the most important person in your life at the moment, the relationship will grow and the trust will build. The only way to communicate this to the patient is to actually feel this way. Make the patient feel comfortable from the start. Each patient who comes in has his own unique problems. To him it may be a major concern...even though to you it may be an everyday occurrence. Don't take it for granted.

Years ago when I was working in an orthopedic office, a woman came rushing through the front door with her seven-year-old son whose arm had just been broken. Although it was a relatively frequent occurrence and something we knew wasn't normally a life or death matter, to her it was a catastrophe. She was panic stricken and fearful for her little boy.

We could have handled it a number of different ways. We could have said, "Your little boy will be fine. Just take a seat and the doctor will see him as soon as he's available." Obviously, this would not have built the relationship, gained any trust, or let the mother and patient know they are important.

Instead, we chose to make the patient and mother feel as though they were the most important people we had at the time. We took them immediately to one of the exam rooms and got the process started. The doctor was informed and he took the few minutes necessary (between his regularly scheduled patients) to speak briefly with the mother and get the order in for the x-ray.

This extra few minutes didn't interrupt the schedule and allowed the mother and little boy to feel like they, and their needs, were important. The next scheduled patients were told of the emergency and were more than happy to wait a few minutes while the child was cared for. They liked the idea that they, too, would get that kind of emergency treatment if they had the need...and they verbally expressed it.

Selling cannot be the responsibility of one member of the team. In many practices the dentist wants to leave the sales part to the rest of the team, or the rest of the team wants to leave it to the doctor, or to the hygienist. But those who do not recognize that the responsibility lies with the entire team will miss incredible opportunities to truly serve the patient and serve the practice as well. Let's first understand and become clear on this one point: There is no "selling part." *It is all selling.* Everything you do is selling: what you say, as well as what you don't say; your body language; everything about you, your team and your practice.

Perhaps you have a treatment coordinator who presents the treatment plan and who does the pre- and post-treatment explanations. And you might feel she is the one who needs to do the selling. And that's fine, she does. Nevertheless, everyone sells, and everyone in the practice should understand the basics of selling.

Because every team member is involved in selling, every person should also be trained. Although it is important that you establish a strong, trusting relationship with the patient, it is just as important for other team members to develop the patient relationship as well. Some patients will tell the assistant, hygienist or receptionist things they won't tell you. Sometimes the patient will look to the auxiliary personnel in making decisions and therefore the team member with great selling skills can be a tremendous asset to the practice. Patient acceptance of treatment will often depend upon the ability of the team member to communicate the benefits of the treatment. Therefore, it is imperative that the team members believe in the practice principles and philosophy. They must understand and believe in the treatment. If they are less than enthusiastic or they don't believe in the treatment, it will be communicated to the patient, either verbally or nonverbally. Remember, we communicate most what we think we communicate least.

Don't prejudge. Doctors sell themselves short by prejudging the patient, by diagnosing what they believe to be the pocketbook capability, or diagnosing based on what insurance will cover, rather than what treatment is truly needed. This is working the treatment plan around your perception of the patients financial status or around the insurance, rather than diagnosing what you believe to be best for the patient. We do this when we look at the appearance or dress of the patient, or the job title, and determine that "I'll have to do a different treatment plan. He'll never accept what I would do for myself (or a family member)."

I can't count the number of times during my years of sales training the number of salespeople who have come up to me during or after a program to say that they pre-judged the customer, lost the sale, and later found that the customer made the "big purchase" somewhere else down the street.

If we say we are really concerned about our patients and their dental health, why don't we present the very best? Usually because we fear rejection. And, as long as we are fearful, that message will be communicated to our patients, non-verbally. The result will often be non-acceptance of the treatment plan, or resistance that takes time to overcome.

We also sell ourselves short when we don't really believe our fees are consistent with the service we offer. Take a moment to think about this. How do you feel about your fees? Do you feel uncomfortable presenting them to the patient? Or do you feel confident, knowing that the value and benefit to the patient equals or exceeds the fee?

> Unless we believe the fee is equal to or less than the value
> of our service to the patient, it will be difficult to feel
> comfortable in presenting the treatment plan and the fees
> attached to it....or to overcome price objections.

Provide value. This may seem obvious, but often when we present treatment plans to our patients *the value isn't clear in their minds.* It is important to remember that much of the dentistry performed today is optional. Certainly you have patients with acute pain and infection, but much treatment today is optional. It becomes clear when we think through this that the competition we are facing is not another dentist, but the shopping centers and malls, vacations, entertainment centers, improvements to homes, new cars, and any number of other "necessities." What has happened is that these other items have become "necessities" in the minds of many, while their dental care becomes the "option." And it is up to us to change that!

The next time you hesitate to present a full treatment plan or the fee that goes with it, remember that this may be the same patient who is eating out several times a week, going to the movies, taking vacations, buying the latest sound technology, purchasing the latest yuppie vehicle, buying more clothes than the closet can hold, etc. There is a perceived value on everything we do and everything we purchase.

> When you and your staff truly believe in
> the value of dentistry...
> and you've put the selling skills into practice...
> you'll see a tremendous difference in your patients'
> acceptance of treatment.

There is an old maxim in sales: we must always remember that the patient is asking (verbally or mentally) WIIFM. What's in it for me? Your patients don't really care what's in it for you. They aren't concerned about your production or your mortgage payment. They don't care if you can take a second or third vacation this year. They want to know what they will get out of the relationship. Again, we need to make the patient feel important and be sure they understand what's in it for them.

Beyond *providing* value, and this goes back to education, we must help our patients *understand* value. Patients will still pay for quality, fee-for-service dentistry if they understand it and it can be related back to their needs, wants and desires. We must take the time to educate each and every patient as to what quality dental health is. If we don't take time to educate them, how will they know?

Selling dentistry requires passion. Is there really any room for lack of passion in our practices? Has anyone succeeded at anything they didn't love? It is difficult to overcome ordinary obstacles and succeed without passion for what you do.

Your Primary Objective

Treatment plan acceptance should be one of the primary objectives of your practice. Everything you do in your dental practice is about having patients accept treatment. That's what you are in business for. It's no fun to examine and diagnose, examine and diagnose, examine and diagnose...and never get to do the treatment! Therefore everything you do, how you speak, what you say, how you behave, the way you listen...everything...should be geared toward treatment plan acceptance.

Because many practitioners are not skilled in selling, when a treatment plan is presented and rejected the "call reluctance" factor sets in. Very simply, that means fear. And the next time it becomes a little more difficult to present the treatment plan for fear of rejection. Enough rejections may lead a dentist to present something less than the optimal, hoping to eliminate a rejection.

> The result of call reluctance is that the
> patients' objections begin to set the standard
> for the dental care you recommend.

Before we move on into the actual selling process, let's remember these two principles:

> *If your patient has a need and you don't present the
> very best possible treatment, you have done your patient
> a disservice.*

> Your patients, every single one of them, should be given
> the opportunity to know about...and either accept
> or reject...the very best care possible.

> *If your patient walks out of the practice without
> necessary treatment completed, they are the loser.*

> If there is necessary work to be done, and you are not
> able to communicate with your patient in such a way
> that he or she understands the importance of the treatment
> and accepts it, then you haven't done your job. The

patient has lost! They aren't getting the care they need. And, of course, you have lost too.

Perfecting your selling skills, and thus the way you present your treatment plans, will yield remarkable rewards. Top producers have this in common. Perhaps no single factor is more important than this. Everything you do must be geared toward the desired ending, and that means selling. Selling is like gardening: you must plant the seeds and then tend to them with the nourishment and care they need in order to get the results you want. And every member of your staff is either nurturing or destroying the process by their attitudes, actions, and words.

When a patient likes the experience of doing business with you, he or she will return again and again.

And that's what sales is all about. The practice, to make this happen, must be patient driven. Everything we do is to help our patients. We must be compassionate and alert to their needs. When we are, they will feel the warmth and kindness, understand our professionalism, trust us, and want to return because they feel good about the experience. It's as simple as that. The only difficult part is carrying it out!

There can be no patient relations without sales. There can be no customer service without sales. There can be no dentistry performed without sales. And there will be no referrals without sales. Every time we are with a patient or talk with a patient over the telephone is a moment of truth, and every moment of truth brings us closer to or pushes us farther away from the sale. Every moment of truth involves your patients making decisions to accept or reject treatment plans, and choosing to remain with your practice or leave for another.

Before we get into the actual process I'd like to share what happened in my husband's dental practice when I began training the staff in sales. We held a half day training session to begin. I briefly did an overview of what the entire selling process is so they could see the big picture. Then we began with the first few steps of The Principled Selling Process and covered them in depth.

Right after the training session our receptionist went back to the office and pulled out some names from her tickler file of people who had not agreed to the treatment plans. Using the tools she had just learned she made the calls and unhesitatingly worked through what she knew of the process. The next day she called me at my office, full of enthusiasm, to tell me she had scheduled four patients whom she felt would never have agreed to the treatment unless she had used the sales principles.

A short time later she came to me again: "These principles really do work, even at home! I'm using them with my children...and they're working!"

It's exciting to know what can happen in a practice when the principles of selling are applied. And it is even more exciting when you begin to see the results!

Success in selling is based on four requirements: obtaining knowledge of the "how" of selling, developing the skills, building and maintaining a positive attitude during the learning curve and beyond, and taking action (implementing those skills).

The Principled Selling process is a *planned approach* to making the sale. It is a "sales track" to run on. When followed, the results will be tremendous. We know that we must begin at the beginning, and work through the process until we get to the close...when we ask the patient for the order, so to speak. Without a process it is hit and miss at best, and when you think you've covered all the essential elements and the patient says no, you don't understand why. The Principled Selling process or "presentation" should appeal to logic and emotion, fit the patient's personality, be constructive, and be presented so it can be understood. When followed, it will lead you to an almost certain yes.

> What you cannot communicate often loses you
> the sale...and therefore controls your practice,
> and as a result, your life.

Therefore, we must plan so we do communicate what we intend to communicate.

The Principled Selling Process is made up of nine steps. Each must be completed in order and you must gain agreement at each step before you go on to the next. These steps are *Prospecting, Making the Approach, Establishing Credibility, Establishing the Need, Presenting the Solution, Closing, Obtaining Referrals, Critiquing the Presentation, and Service (follow-up).*

Remember: ***A sale is a value judgment arrived at in the mind of a person (a prospective patient or current patient) with the ability to buy.*** It's a decision about what you have to offer, and that's where the education comes in. Many people don't understand their need when it comes to dentistry. It is our job as healthcare professionals to help them understand. That means beginning at the beginning, being patient, and realizing that many have never had the basis of knowledge with which to understand the importance of homecare and dentistry. Remember Fred's story. Remember my story.

I grew up in a family that was involved in medicine. I was quite aware of my own health and preventive measures to maintain good health. I also thought I was quite aware of dental health. I had regular check-ups and I accepted the dentistry I was told needed to be done.

It wasn't until I married Norm that I learned about many home-care issues...and no one had ever told me about flossing (even though I had worked in a dental office many years before)! I wasn't educated.

Unfortunately, many people never really understand how important their natural teeth are until they don't have them. Then, it's too late. How are you doing in educating your patients? If they aren't educated, and don't understand, your chances of having the treatment plan accepted "just because the doctor said so" will be far less than desired.

One other factor is involved here. Many people see dentistry as elective. Without selling skills it is highly likely that you might be experiencing (or will in the future) lowered treatment plan acceptance and production problems. Good selling skills will help you maximize treatment acceptance with every patient. You'll get more yeses to needed treatment and when that happens, you won't need as many patients! It is much more difficult, time consuming, and expensive to continually market in order to have a large enough number of new patients that, even with a lower "closing" ratio, will give enough accepted dentistry to keep the practice alive.

There is a paradox at work here. Although people in this country are more health conscious today than ever before, it doesn't necessarily mean they are doing what is best for themselves. And, although many people say they want to be involved with their medical/dental issues and be a part of the process rather than having "it" just done to them, many deep down still don't want to be responsible for their health. If there was a magic formula for doing something once and being done with dentistry for the rest of their lives, many would certainly jump on the bandwagon. But we are dealing with human nature and habits, and it takes time to change those habits...even when a person is completely willing.

What this means for us is that we must go slowly and develop trust. And, as we see minor changes in the direction we want our patients to move, we must praise them for the good they are doing.

For example, you have a new patient who needs $5,000 of restorative work. This patient, however, has neglected dental health and general physical health for years, has periodontal disease, and has not visited a dentist regularly. It is doubtful that you will be able to convince him after one appointment that he needs to deal with the perio problems and go ahead with the $5,000 of restorative treatment. This person, more than likely, will need to be brought around slowly. He needs to be educated deliberately, consistently and completely, and then you'll have greater success in bringing him around.

Building trust is one of the great principles of The Principled Selling Process and is built into each step. Let's take a look at the process in depth. Here's where the rubber hits the pavement. Learn this process, begin applying it, and you'll realize incredible results. Steps one (prospecting)and eight (critiquing the presentation) do not involve the patients directly...they involve you. The other seven steps, however, involve the patient fully.

Chapter 24

STEP 1: PROSPECTING

Prospecting is the first step in the process. Defined, it is *the search for and identification of qualified buyers of your dental services.* Qualified buyers are identified by the acronym MAPS:

Money (they have the ability to buy)
Authority (they can make the decision to buy, or can
    gain the agreement of the decision maker
Problem (they have a need, want, or desire)
Seen (they can be seen on a favorable basis)

If the prospective patient does not meet these four requirements, gaining treatment acceptance will be next to impossible. It is imperative that we understand these four factors that constitute a qualified buyer. Otherwise, we may end up wasting time on a person we think is a prospect but who is really a china egg. And china eggs don't hatch!

Has the money to purchase your services. The prospective patient must be capable of producing the funds to purchase your services. He may not have the funds readily available to pay cash up front, but unless he can meet whatever financial options you make available (such as Visa, Master Card, various healthcare credit cards, etc.) or have the ability to obtain a loan, or you choose to work out financial arrangements they can carry out, then again you don't have a prospect. You're providing a service and you have every right to expect payment for those services.

Has the authority to buy. Unless you intend to do free dentistry, this is certainly a must for a qualified prospect. This means that the person has the authority to make the decision, or can get that authority from the decision maker to purchase your dental services. No matter how great the need, or how much money a person has, if you can't get past this one, you don't have a qualified prospect. You have a china egg.

Has a problem (need, want, desire). Many people who come into your practice probably don't understand the need for the treatment you've outlined. In fact, if the tooth or teeth are asymptomatic they may even question your proposal! That's where the educational process comes in. We'll discuss this fully in chapter twenty-seven. Nevertheless, the patient must have a need, want or desire. If none of the three exist, you don't have a qualified prospective patient.

Can be seen on a favorable basis. This is one factor many people don't know about, or if they do, they forget about. Sometimes you'll meet a person you just can't seem to connect with. No matter how hard you try, you just seem to butt heads and meet with friction at every turn. These are usually the patients who cause the bulk of your frustration and concern in your practice. And you do have a choice. You don't have to accept these individuals as patients. If you cannot see someone on a favorable basis, getting them to accept dentistry may prove to be a major chore.

Many people in "sales" positions cry out, "My trouble isn't selling...I can sell. My trouble is prospecting...I can't find people to sell." Prospecting itself needs to become a *process*. Prospects are like a short term bank account requiring daily withdrawals, therefore needing daily deposits. Every day you complete dentistry on a patient...and unless that individual develops additional problems, there is no further work to be done except the regular hygiene and check-ups. Patients will die, move away, choose to go to another dentist even though they don't move, or leave because they are dissatisfied. That means you must continually add new patients. Great selling skills will help you get more dentistry accepted and therefore you won't need as many new patients as you would otherwise.

In the marketing section we covered numerous sources of prospects. Again, the key to prospecting is to make it a system, a process. When it becomes a process it no longer becomes a problem. Choose what methods you will use to find your new patients. Don't try everything on the list; that would be virtually impossible to do and it will give you mental indigestion! Choose a few methods you feel will work well in your practice, and then cultivate those sources regularly. When you do you will have a continual flow of new prospective patients into your practice.

It is important to understand that just because a person shows up in your practice for a new patient exam, it doesn't mean they have become your patient. Technically, yes. But until they return for another appointment or two, you can't really consider them a regular patient. If they only show up once they haven't done much for themselves, and they haven't added much value to the practice.

Remember your profile. Who are you looking for? What is your prospective patient profile. You'll need to clearly identify this to make your prospecting process work for you. Once you have identified your prospect sources, you are ready to take the next step.

Chapter 25

STEP II: MAKING THE APPROACH

The approach, defined as *the first contact with your prospective patient,* is the second step of the Principled Selling process. Whether it be on the telephone or in person, you want the prospective patient conditioned to respond favorably to you, your staff, and your recommendation of treatment. Every time the patient is introduced to another person in the practice, another approach is made. Perception is everything here. Patients *will* judge. They will make their decisions about how they feel about you, the staff, and the practice based on their perception. When you or any of your team members meet a patient, does your behavior inspire trust? The likability factor and a smile is important here. Darwin said, "If a smile doesn't produce crows feet at the corners of the eyes, it doesn't read as fully felt."

Think about all the approaches that are made. The front desk person makes an approach over the telephone and in person. The assistant usually makes the next approach. The next might be the doctor and then the hygienist. Every single person makes an approach to the patient, and every time it is either building up or tearing down the patient's perception of the practice. How we greet our patients is critically important; every action is building your image and affecting your credibility. Every team member is responsible for representing your practice.

Sometimes we make a mistake here: we forget about the importance of the first impression. Remember, you never get a second chance to make a first impression. Those first few seconds are vitally important. It will take a long time (if you're even given the opportunity) to reverse a negative first impression. Some simple guidelines here will help.

First, be yourself. People feel uncomfortable when they feel other people are uncomfortable. Be yourself, but be your best self.

Many years ago as a sales manager for a national insurance company, I was asked to conduct a training session at another office for new agents, and discuss the basics of the sales process. I spoke about being yourself in the approach. When the session was over one gentlemen who had been in the business for eleven months came up to me and said:

Thank you. You don't know what you've just done for me. You see, I have felt, for some reason, that I had to be somebody other than myself in order to be a true professional. I never knew it was okay to be myself. And, quite frankly, if someone would have told me this early in my training, maybe I wouldn't have had to suffer the eleven months of hell I've gone through trying to be someone other than me. Thank you. I'm sure this business will be a lot more fun now.

Second, put yourself in your patient's shoes. What is the typical attitude here? Most likely he will be a bit wary or on guard. He doesn't know you and he's not sure he can trust you. He may be a bit apprehensive because he doesn't have confidence (yet) and he doesn't want to be "sold." That's only natural. Until you and your team give the patient a reason to think and feel otherwise, that's that way it is.

Third, tune out the world and tune in the prospect. Give the patient your full attention. Pay attention to your eye contact. "Listen" to how he feels. Treat each person as the *person* they are, with feelings, ambitions, fears, concerns, etc...not as an *object*. Too often people are treated as numbers or objects...and they don't like it. They want to be treated as individuals with their own unique feelings, desires, wants, and ambitions. Each patient will respond differently, and will send out clues to tell you who and where they are, if you'll ask questions and care enough to listen. Part of your professionalism and selling ability depends upon how well you pick-up and process those clues. When you are with a patient that is not the time to be thinking about the last patient you saw, or the one coming in next. It's not the time to be thinking about your golf game that evening or where you're going on vacation in two weeks. It's time to give the patient your full attention. Make him feel as though he is the most important person in the world to you at that time. And you can't give that feeling unless that's how you really feel. When you're with that patient, he *is* your world at that moment.

Fourth, always put the patient first. This means get the patient talking about himself. Ask non threatening questions, then relax and listen. By being relaxed you'll help the prospect relax. The best way to relax is to take the focus off yourself. Don't be wondering what the patient is thinking about you or your team, or how you're going to proceed next. Put your focus on the patient; listen and really be there for that patient.

Fifth, have fun and smile. Let the patient know you like what you do and you're glad he's there (or on the phone with you) by the way you communicate with him.

Sixth, believe that you are on the way to building a solid, lasting, healthy, accepting relationship with this patient. Again, remember that we communicate most what we think we're communicating least. Patients pick-up on your feelings. They will know if you are feeling a lack of confidence. They'll know if you really wish they weren't there. They'll know if the only thing you're thinking about is getting out of the office. They'll know if you're thinking "you're a turkey." And they'll know that about every team member! They may not be able to verbalize it as such, but they'll know something "doesn't feel quite right."

When you first meet the patient, begin building rapport by asking general questions. Get the patient talking. Perhaps he was referred by another patient of yours (and you should know this before you see the patient). To initiate the conversation you might say, *"I understand Tom Smith referred you to our practice. How do you know Tom?"* Or you might say, *"I understand Tom referred you to our practice. Are you an avid golfer like Tom ?"*

An easy way to make sure you will have something to begin building on is to ask a couple questions on your patient information or history form that you can use. For example, include a question as to "Who may we thank for referring you?" Or you might ask "What hobbies or activities do you participate in?" It doesn't take much, but being able to ask a relevant question of the patient will help break the ice and begin building rapport.

When you ask any salesperson what the most difficult part of selling is, many will tell you closing. Actually, this is not the case at all. The most difficult part of selling is making the approach because it is here that you establish the tone of the relationship. When you are successful in the approach the next step can flow naturally and smoothly.

Gain Agreement

It's important to point out here that agreement must be gained throughout the entire selling process, beginning with the approach. When you have followed The Principled Selling Process all the way through with a patient, you should already know by the time you ask the final question whether or not the patient will be going ahead with the treatment. That's how the process is designed. By gaining agreement at every step, and several times in each step, you will know whether or not you can proceed.

> Gaining agreement means getting the patient
> to say yes, nod their head, or to show agreement
> by some form of affirmation.

A good rule of thumb here is to continually take the temperature of the patient by summarizing every three to four sentences or at least at the end of a thought sequence and gain the agreement.

It sounds as though you've had an uncomfortable experience with dentistry somewhere in the past, is that true? Could you tell me about it?

After the explanation...*I'm sorry to hear about that. Things have changed a lot in dentistry over the past few years, and I'm sure you'll find the new equipment and procedures to be remarkably different from what you've just described to me. That will be pleasant change for you, won't it?*

When you gain the agreement you are checking to make sure the patient is still with you, that you are both on the same track, and that you've understood the patient.

So you've moved here from the East Coast and you were referred to our office by your next door neighbor? That's great, and we're very pleased you've selected our practice for your dental needs. We'll do everything we can to make your association with us a great experience. Sound fair enough?

Three Rules in the Presentation

Before we move on, there are three rules which should be adhered to throughout the entire presentation.

1. Never argue. Discuss, but never argue. You may win the argument but lose the sale, so to speak.
2. Never preach or talk down to a patient. People don't like to feel they are being preached "at" or talked "down to." They want to be a part of the process.
3. Never tell a patient what he or she should do...rather, suggest or recommend. We'll talk about how to do this later, but recognize that today people want to take part in their healthcare. Some may still accept the"should's," but many more won't. Therefore, move away from the "should's" so you won't offend anyone, and thus possibly lose a patient or treatment acceptance.

Also, it is important that we not put a patient on the defensive at any time during their visit to your practice. Patients are good at defending their positions; if you both are put in the position of defending, most often you and the practice will lose.

Chapter 26

STEP III: ESTABLISHING CREDIBILITY

The principle that comes into play here is: *People don't care how much you know until they know how much you care.* Establishing credibility involves creating an atmosphere for successful selling. It means gaining the confidence of the patient and building trust. Before you sell anything to a patient, any treatment plan, you must first begin to establish a safe, trusting relationship.

Strong relationships are built on a foundation of communication that includes listening, understanding, responding and interacting, and subsequently leads to trust. To be credible, what we say and what we do must be congruent.

Until you have the trust and confidence of your patients, they will never follow your direction, purchase your services, or "buy" you as their dentist. They may follow through with their initial appointment because they don't feel comfortable leaving in the middle of it, but they may not return. People want the kind of attention that says, "You are important; we care about you; we're here to help you; and we love being of service to you." Because this is so vital, the new patient experience in our practices must be a great one.

How do you establish that trust? Every person must be well trained in their job responsibilities and come across to the patient as knowledgeable, professional and competent. Every team member must have the energy of passion and enthusiasm for what they do. The patient will know if it is there...and they will know if it isn't! Every team member must show by their actions that they care. This means they must be truly "present" to the patient when they are with the patient. Every step of the patient's journey through your practice must be handled with attention to detail, from the first phone call all the way through the first appointment, as well as at every subsequent appointment. Unless our patients see us this way, they will have at least one reason to search for another practice. Remember this acronym that is helpful in building credibility:

ISECADA
Interest, Sincerity, Enthusiasm Create A Desired Atmosphere

At this stage in the selling process the patient should be curious and interested. The buying decision the patient has to make here is that he wants to do business with you; he wants to seriously consider your recommendation. He is making the decision here as to whether or not he will listen to what you have to say.

Your job as the "salesperson" is to help the patient feel secure and gain agreement that "Yes, you are a good person to do business with and your practice is where I want to have my dentistry completed."

As you begin to establish credibility, give the patient reasons to do business with you. Think through what you will say and how you will say it. Write it down, actually script it out. Unless you do you will be changing it every time you speak to a new patient. Perhaps you'll want to share some of the following with your patient:

- How long you've been in practice.
- Your credentials (and those of your staff)
- Why you are practicing dentistry (to let them know you love it!)

- Practice philosophy (optimum dental health, caring, concern, warmth, etc.)
- Track record (on time for appointments, quality of dentistry, etc.)
- What you will do for your patient (your commitment to the patient)
- What makes you different from other dental offices (without putting down others in the process)

Other questions in addition to the above, that patients will have in their minds, consciously or subconsciously, are:

- Are you sincere?
- How will you handle any emergency I might have?
- Will you not talk down to me or belittle me?
- Will you listen to my needs and my questions?
- Will you allow me to ask questions?
- Will you be gentle...and minimize any pain?
- Do you care about me as an individual?
- Are you friendly, courteous?
- Do you value my time?
- How safe will I be?
- Is your equipment state-of-the-art?
- Do you stay up on the most current technology and methods, as well as materials?
- Will you help me be able to afford my treatment (financial options)?

Any and all of these points can be used to establish your credibility and your practice as a good place for the patient to be. As you talk about each one, however, make sure you remember the WIIFM. What's in it for me? Patients are interested in these points only to the extent that they are benefits for them. Make the connection for your patients. For example:

Our practice philosophy is to provide every patient with the opportunity for optimum dental health in a warm, caring environment. This means you can count on us to always recommend treatment that is in your very best interests, and that is important to you, isn't it?

Notice how the question at the end gains the agreement, as well as builds the credibility. Remember to gain agreement all the way through the entire process. If the patient says, "Yes, it is" then you've just moved one step closer to the sale. Here's another example:

Most often we are right on schedule for your appointment and we strive to maintain that record because we value your time. This allows you to plan your day better and maximize your effectiveness. Would you say that's a benefit that you would enjoy?

Again, build credibility and at the same time gain agreement.

It is important to invest the time, at least a few minutes, building your credibility with your patients by helping them to understand the benefits of being with you in your practice.

Everything *you* do, and everything your *team members* do,
is either building credibility or tearing it down.

Further, you can build your credibility by third party influence. Testimonials by your patients are an example of this. Place them in a "show and tell" book in the reception area. Tie in before and after pictures with the testimony of your patient along side (be sure to get permission before you use testimonials and pictures of your patients). Unsolicited letters from patients are also a great credibility builder to at least begin the process before the patient has had much experience with you or your team. Here's an example of such a letter received recently in our practice.

Dear Dr. Matschek,
As a new patient to your office, I could not be more pleased with my initial experience. This attitude is expressed towards your manner and procedures as well as that of your office staff.
I feel is important that someone in your position be well educated and trained in his field. However, I feel it is equally important that he possess the skills that enable him to relay

this to the patient in a confident but personable manner. I would like to express my appreciation to you for providing both of these qualities at my June 20 visit.

So often patients, the public in general, make the time to comment when things are below acceptable standards, so I just wanted to let you and your staff know that I greatly appreciate your "above and beyond" service!

Sincerely,
Chris D. (patient)

Once you've spent a little time in establishing your credibility and you've gained agreement from the patient that what you have to offer is important to him, then you can move to the next step of the selling process from a position of strength.

Chapter 27

STEP IV: IDENTIFYING THE NEED

The technical quality of care has improved tremendously in medicine and dentistry over the years, but there is a growing feeling that we are losing something very important...the careful listening and empathic responding by the healthcare provider. According to the results of several surveys, patients have little to complain about concerning the competence and expertise of their healthcare providers, but they are dissatisfied with the human element. They want the opportunity to talk, to be listened to, and to be told as much as possible, but frequently this doesn't happen. Even when the doctor does relay clinical information, it is useless if the patients can't understand it. The need identification stage is a great place to bring this back home.

We need to be attentive not only to the health and function of our patient's mouths, but to their desire to look and feel the best they can. This is a major change for dentists who have been trained to diagnose pathology and then tell patients what treatment is needed. Today, the doctor must learn to relate the diagnosed treatment to what the patient wants. This requires a whole new set of skills. Patients are motivated by their own desires and we must communicate with that in mind.

Understanding the patient's needs, values, fears and goals is necessary in order to sell our dental services effectively. We must learn to see through the eyes of our patients, through their experiences, and step into their shoes until we have a good understanding of their situation *from their perspective.* In sales, we must *focus on the benefits to the patient,* and we cannot do this without knowing what is a benefit to them. And, it is only a benefit if it is perceived as one! That is the objective of the next two selling steps.

Education is the first step to help patients understand and then turn that understanding into a want or desire for the dentistry. So often it is the uneducated patients (in all aspects of the practice) that ends up unhappy with the result.

So how do we go about doing this? This is what identifying the need, want or desire is all about. The only way to do this is to ask questions...then listen. A good sales presentation is a discovery process, not a speech. And it is no less in dentistry. If you encounter resistance when you present the treatment plan, or when you meet with an objection or a stall, often it is because this step of the sales process was not completed. You must have a well-defined sense of where the patient is and what he wants before you can present the solution...the treatment plan.

The attitude of the patient at this point should be curious. He has come this far with you, has heard about why this is a good place to be, and now is ready to test it out.

> The buying decision the patient has to make in the
> need identification stage of the selling process is that he
> has a problem to be solved, or a need, want, or desire
> to be filled.

In this stage of the selling process you want to *intensify* his interest, *disturb* the patient, and *gain agreement* that he has a problem, need, want or desire.

Before any solution can be presented, the patient must come to see and fully agree that he or she has a problem to be solved. We can present information to a patient, but most people will not act simply on information. *The information needs to move the patient to thinking...and then to feeling.*

We buy on emotion and
back it up with logic.

To move from the informational stage to the feeling stage, you must intensify the patient's interest...you must *disturb* the patient. That may sound a bit harsh, but it is extremely important. Unless the patient is disturbed and really feels and believes the need is there, he probably won't be motivated to do anything about it. If we are not disturbed, we will have virtually no reason to "move to action."

A young traveling salesman wrote on his weekly report to his sales manager that he had called on 40 prospective buyers during the past week, but after getting them to the edge of the water he couldn't make them drink.

His manager replied, "Whoever told you your job is to make them drink? All you have to do is make them thirsty!"

That's what we want to do with our patients; to make them thirsty for what they need, as well as what they want. The thirst is the disturbance. To do this you must get the patient involved. Many attempts to get the patient involved boil down to a tremendous effort to talk *to* the patient, rather than *with* the patient.

Selling isn't telling; it is listening,
asking questions, and listening again.

It has been said that God gave us two ears and one mouth and that we should use them in that proportion! Drowning the patient in a sea of facts about their dental health won't necessarily establish the need and disturb the patient enough to move him to action. Learn to ask questions, and listen. Trust cannot be built without listening. Probe the patient about his wishes, desires, needs, problems, concerns and objectives. Let the patient talk. Hear what the patient is saying, as well as what he is not saying. When you are talking you are learning very little about what is going on inside the patient. When the patient is talking and responding to your well directed questions, you will learn a great deal. Most important, you will learn what the patient is interested in and bothered by, and that is precisely what will allow you to move the patient to accept the treatment you diagnose. The talking you do should be directed...that is, using questions you have already thought about and committed to memory to focus the direction of the conversation.

Perhaps you think you don't need to ask the patient many questions, that you'll find out what you need to know by doing the examination and taking radiographs. But if you don't ask questions to find out *what is important to your patient,* you may never be able to get the agreement to go ahead with the treatment plan you present. Even when you know immediately what the situation is and you know the patient's needs, don't tell...ask ! And when he tells you, he'll believe it!

> **When you ask questions and listen,**
> **your integrity is perceived as much greater.**

The patient feels cared for and can sense your genuine interest.

In other words, if your patient is interested primarily in "looks," in order to disturb him or move him emotionally so he will make a positive decision to accept treatment when you relate your findings, it is important that you tie your proposed treatment into his appearance. Or, perhaps your patient is very health conscious and wants to do everything possible to maintain his good health. When you relate your diagnosis to him with the proposed treatment, he will respond much more readily if you relate the treatment needs to his health.

Regardless of what *you* believe or feel, if the *patient* doesn't believe and feel it, the likelihood of acceptance decreases dramatically.

In the need identification stage of selling, you are fact-finding. You've always done that from a clinical standpoint, but it is important to add the psychological fact finding as well. What is important to your patient? Find this out before you begin the clinical fact-finding. You'll find much greater treatment plan acceptance at the end, and you'll also find a much more willing patient to go through the diagnostic steps necessary to get to that end.

Buying Motives

It is helpful to understand why people buy. Basically the buying motives are:

- Vanity or pride (cosmetics, looks, how they compare with others, etc.)
- Profit (will save money by acting now rather than waiting until later...greater problems with bigger price tags may result by waiting)
- Security (peace of mind, freedom from loss, not wanting to lose teeth, don't want dentures)
- Personal gain (freedom from pain, improvement, self-image enhancement, better health)
- Love

People don't buy what they need unless it is also what they want. You can tell them, show them pictures, tell them about other patients in the same situation all day long, and still not get the commitment for their dentistry. Only when you can relate what is needed to something they want will you gain their commitment.

Setting the Stage

When you first see your patient, introduce yourself (or have your assistant introduce you to the patient), sit down and take the time to talk. Get to know the patient, as well as what the patient thinks he wants. Remember, they don't care how much you know until they know how much you care. So you have a busy schedule and don't believe you can take this time? What good does it do to race through your day, see large numbers of patients, not take the time to build the relationship, and have a low acceptance ratio of treatment plans in the end?

Second, approach dentistry from the total person approach. We're not simply treating the mouth of the patient. Improving esthetics will improve the way the patient feels about him or herself, their security, the way they relate to other people, the way they chew and function.

Third, if this is a cosmetic patient, consider asking that patient to have someone who has influence on them (spouse, relative, friend) to come to the office in the planning stages. This will diminish the possibility of the patient coming back and being unhappy because family or friends don't like the "look." A good example of this happened to one of my clients.

The patient was in her sixties, and was quite active in the higher social circles of her home town. She wanted to have her entire mouth reconstructed with veneers and went ahead with the treatment. Following completion, she was elated with the result. But that quickly changed.

She went home and was surprised to find that her husband didn't at all like the result. He was actually angry with her for having it done, and began threatening a lawsuit.

It is important for the patient to understand that functional dental health is critical to the success of cosmetic improvements. Discuss the status of their dental health, changes that might need to be made, and specialists they may need to see before cosmetic treatment is begun.

Satisfaction in the end will greatly depend
upon how involved the patient was in making
the decision in the beginning.

The Use of Questions in Need Identification

Open ended questions will give you the greatest amount of information. These are the essay type questions that get the patient involved and participating in the discovery process to help you uncover his wants, needs and desires, as well as lead you into the clinical fact-finding that will follow. In the early stages of working with a patient open-ended questions are preferable.

Open ended questions often begin with *what, how,* and *would you tell me. Why* is sometimes appropriate, but caution is needed here. When we begin a question with "why" people often feel put on the defensive. Occasionally *who, where* and *when* are appropriate, but they approximate the closed-ended questions.

Using these closed-ended questions requires asking too many questions in rapid succession to gain the same information you could otherwise get from open-ended questions. They also sound like the "third degree" or "list of twenty questions." Remember, when you ask questions you must listen to and concentrate on the patient and what he is saying, not on what you are going to say or ask next. When you give your full attention you will gain valuable information and hear many clues to the patient's hot buttons.

An example of a closed-ended question, better replaced with an open-ended one, is this:

Closed: Do you have pain at night?
Open: When do you usually feel or experience pain?

Obviously the possibility for more information comes with the open-ended question. Closed-ended questions are particularly useful in the later stages of the selling process. They risk a no response, however, and are usually used to confirm needs. They are also appropriate when you want to limit the range of the patient's response to a yes or no, or when you want to ask a choice question. *Do, are, which, has, is, have,* and *does* are all openings for closed-ended questions.

Questions not only get the patient involved, but they actually *focus* the patient's thinking, *create disturbance* as the patient begins to see the need or problem unfold, *enable you to ask* your patient's opinions or feelings, *identify areas of interest,* and *save you time* in the long run. They practically guarantee acceptance of your treatment plan if done well. They give the patient the opportunity to see his own dental needs in a different light. And when the patient tells you his or her concerns, you don't have to fight to get him to accept your ideas and treatment plan because you've related them back to his hot buttons. Done the other way, *telling* patients what they need, can put them on the defensive and cause resistance to your treatment recommendations.

I call this the SNAQ approach...smile, nod and ask questions. In other words, be friendly, encourage your patient to continue talking and responding to you (by nodding) and ask questions to identify needs, wants, desires and concerns. Remember ISECADA (interest, sincerity, enthusiasm create a desired atmosphere).

Throughout the need identification stage, remember that one of the best ways to learn about your patient is to use the golden pause at two points in your questioning. First, after you have asked the question, and second, after the patient has answered. The golden pause is a 2-3 second pause that will benefit you and the patient. People don't always respond right away. Many need the time to ingest, think, digest, and analyze before they respond. When you allow the pause, you will get more responses and they will be more comprehensive. Your patient will feel more comfortable when you give them time to think about and consider their responses. Another benefit of the pause is that you have just given yourself permission to be totally present with the patient as he or she speaks...not thinking of what you are going to say next, but really listening. You can use your pause time to consider your comments or questions after giving the patient your full, undivided attention. As a result, your response will be more relevant because you listened.

Here are a variety of open-ended questions that may be helpful to you in the need identification stage:

- If you could change anything you wanted about your smile, what would it be?
- How do you see your mouth in ten (twenty) years?
- How important is it for you to keep your teeth for your lifetime?
- If we can help you keep your teeth all your life, how important would that be to you?
- What is it about keeping your teeth that is important to you?
- What does dental health mean to you?
- How happy are you with the color of your teeth?
- How important is it to you to prevent dental emergencies for yourself?
- How important is your smile to your career?
- If you could change anything about your teeth, what would it be?
- How helpful would it be for you to have as few dental treatment visits as possible?

- If there was a way to have 90% of the dental treatment for the rest of your life completed now, how interested would you be?
- How long have you had this swelling?

As you gather information and begin to gain an understanding of your patients wants and desires, you may want to use a few well-directed, closed-ended questions to get at any specifics you want answered, such as:

- When you look in the mirror at your teeth, is there anything you see that you would like to be different?
- Is there anything about your smile or appearance of your teeth that you don't like and would like to change if it were possible?
- Do you snore?
- Do you have any missing teeth? Have they been replaced? Is it fixed or can you remove it? Is it working well for you?
- Do you have any particular concerns about your dental health or dental treatment that you would like to discuss?
- When was the last time we talked about this? (Used when an existing patient has not accepted the treatment that was diagnosed some time ago.)

We want to get the patient involved as much as possible and that's what the need identification step is designed to do. When you do have the patient involved you will build a stronger, more solid relationship with that patient, and you will have a higher level of acceptance.

The need identification stage of the selling process calls forth the very best of your communication skills. Problems can arise because we listen selectively; we anticipate where the patient is going with their thoughts and jump in before we really know. We need to ask questions and then listen closely to all that is said, and what is not said. We need to disturb the patient. Make sure you don't wait until you are ready to present the treatment plan to disturb the patient. It must develop during the dialogue and examination process. If it isn't, most likely it will be difficult to get the patient to a level of emotional discomfort and disturbance when you present the treatment plan.

Ask questions throughout the need identification stage and paraphrase the response back to the patient to make sure you understand. When you do this you set the stage for acceptance of the solution which comes next. Here are six examples:

Mrs. Jones, what I hear you telling me is that you've never been happy with your smile because of the space between your teeth? Is that correct?

Let me make sure I understand you correctly. Your smile and your appearance is very important to you. You're in a business that requires a lot of personal communication and you want to do everything possible to make sure you keep your teeth for your lifetime. Is that correct?

Let's see if I understand exactly what you're telling me. You've had what you consider to be a bad dental experience and you're hesitant to make any decisions now, which is why you've put off a dental exam. But you are concerned about your total health and you know something is not right because your gums bleed and a number of teeth are somewhat loose. Is this correct?

Just so I'm clear on what you're really looking for, you want (and then name what they've indicated their hot button is). Is that correct?

Based on what you just told me, your immediate concern is (name what you have identified as their hot button). Is that right?

What I hear you saying is that you want (paraphrase what they have indicated is important to them). Am I correct?

A key point to remember here is this: **Don't tell people things you can ask them.** When you ask and they respond, you can then paraphrase and gain agreement. But if you tell, you may never know if they agree. When you ask the questions and they tell you, they believe it. Remember that as you ask questions you must be enthusiastic, aware, and tuned into your patient.

Each one of these questions sets the stage for you to go on. The question at the end of your paraphrasing is a "tie down." Their affirmative response *ties down* the statement in question. It "nails down" their agreement that they have a problem, need, want, or desire. All the time you are asking questions, remember the SNAQ approach. Smile and nod yes as you ask the question.

Selling is a participation and involvement process...not a spectator sport performed by the patient. And again, the way to get the patient involved is to ask questions, listen, and then gain agreement.

Now, whatever the patient agrees to in the need identification stage of the selling process you can refer to later in the solution. Once you have asked your questions and are sufficiently comfortable that you have begun the process of getting to know your patient and his hot buttons, it is time to do the clinical exam.

Before we go on to the exam, however, there is another point where it is important we ask a few specific questions. Questioning the patient before beginning treatment (at the time of every appointment) is also helpful:

> *Do you have any questions about what we are going to be doing for you today?*

Ask this before you have the patient lying back...and when you are at eye level with the patient. Ask in a manner that shows no hurry, stress, or tension. It is important to make sure the patient is relaxed, comfortable, and doesn't have questions before you begin treatment.

Effective questioning is an art that must be practiced until you can do it well and effectively. Asking questions that get to the heart of the matter requires feeling, enthusiasm, vitality and aliveness, deep conviction and certainly knowledge of dentistry.

Completing the Exam

The clinical examination is the second part of the need identification process. Before you begin the exam, talk with your patient about what you are going to do and why. Here is another great time to build credibility. Explain what a comprehensive examination involves and why. As you walk through the exam, talk to your patient about what you are doing and finding, for example:

As you check the neck and glands for enlargements or irregularities, don't stop at just telling the patient that "I'm checking your neck and glands." Don't leave the translation up to the patient. Tell them why you are checking and what you are checking for.

Or another example, "Let me show you some important things about your mouth." Then begin by showing what healthy tissue looks like (hopefully there is some!) "This is what healthy tissue looks like. " As you proceed using the probe, "This is 2 mm...and that's healthy. If you keep all your teeth and gums this healthy you'll most likely keep your teeth as long as you live."

Continue probing and show what is normal, good, etc. But when the probe drops:

I want to show you something. Look at this. You're developing a problem here. It may not be a problem yet....(as you probe and pus oozes out). See this pus. It is caused by tissue breaking down. I don't know what is causing this, but there is nothing more important for me to do at this time than to find out. A pocket like this won't clean itself out or cure itself. What I want to do today is find out what is going on and determine what we can do to stop it. If it continues, it can lead to tooth loss.

Perhaps you come to an area where there is substantial plaque build-up. Again, explain what is going on and create word pictures.

Can you see this area? This is what is called plaque. Plaque is live germs...and what it does is create an acid that etches into the tooth causing decay. When I clean the plaque away can you see how it is etched and chalky? And over here the healthy tooth structure is clean and shining?

We'll work with you to help you learn how to keep your teeth and gums really clean and healthy. There is no reason you can't keep your teeth for your lifetime if we begin right away....before it is too late. And you did say that's important to you, didn't you?

After you make the entire trip around the patient's mouth, show him wthere are problems and where there are no problems, where there are fractures, where amalgams are breaking down, where there is inflammation, plaque, etc. Also compliment the patient on what you see that is good and well taken care of. Most of all, don't talk down to the patient through this process, or use a tone of voice that is condemning, disgusting, or judgmental. Let your patients know by your words and your actions that you accept them, and that you are there to diagnose the situation and help them do what is necessary to restore their mouth to good dental health.

Intraoral Cameras

The number one reason people don't go to the dentist or accept a treatment plan is lack of dental education. That's what this entire Principled Selling process is designed to do...educate patients.

Eighty-three percent of a person's learning takes place visually, and therein lies the secret of the intraoral camera, *if it is used effectively and often.* There is an old maxim in training: Tell me and I will be sure to forget; show me and I might remember or understand; get me involved and I will understand and follow-through.

The intraoral cameras and imaging systems have provided us with a tremendous opportunity to foster the educational experience. They actually enhance the dentist's and hygienist's communication with the patients and shorten the amount of time it takes to get the message across so the patients understand it.

> People don't buy what they need...
> they buy what they want.

You can tell them, show them pictures, tell them about other patients all day, and still not get the commitment for their dentistry. When you show them via an intraoral camera, the need becomes apparent. The patient's response is phenomenal when these cameras are used correctly. Patients can understand a comprehensive treatment plan much better when the image on the screen is

sive treatment plan much better when the image on the screen is them rather than a model or picture in a book or brochure. The visual image allows the patient to see and understand, which helps in making decisions easier, faster, and with more confidence. When patients truly understand their needs, they can become wants, and then they will buy.

Psychologically there is nothing as potent and effective for your patients as seeing themselves on a color monitor as you educate them about their condition. With the intraoral camera, you can create a color print of their mouth and give it to them as part of their education process. It provides a new avenue for discussion between you and your patient. Often, in the past, discussion has been left out of the treatment plan proposal. It was a one-sided process...a monologue. As we've already seen, unless the patient is involved, it will be difficult to raise the patient's emotional level to disturbance, and thus it will be much more difficult to gain acceptance of the treatment plan.

The intraoral camera and imaging system brings dentistry to a new level of understanding for the lay person. If you have an intraoral camera it will be most effective and get you the greatest results when it is used continuously in your practice. It can be used with every new patient and with every hygiene patient, and with other patients as appropriate. If it is, it will become a profit center, not an overhead factor. Maximizing the benefits you can receive from your intraoral camera requires a commitment by you and your hygienist or other trained staff member to use it at every possible appointment. If you don't have an intraoral camera, it may be a wise decision to investigate the benefits for your practice. It won't be long before it will become a regular part of every practice, and patients will be asking for it. The use of these cameras allows you to offer a level of education that creates the desire and disturbance on the part of the patient for dental treatment. When used properly, patients will literally be *asking you* what can be done and how soon they can get it done.

It is critical that the entire team understand that a patient must be educated, disturbed, and emotionally involved before they can request or accept treatment. The intraoral camera is a great way to better educate your patients about their problems, and it contributes to a positive experience. When patients understand their needs the work you do and the service you and your team provide. Whether it is a new or existing patient, the intraoral camera is a great communication device. By using the intraoral camera properly and often, you can get your patients to "own" their dental problems and "emotionally buy into them," thus moving them closer to acceptance of the necessary treatment.

Our treatment plans need to become persuasive rather than simply informative. When we do, we will find fewer and fewer patients walking out the door unscheduled, and not accepting treatment. Word pictures created in the mind of the patient will help us to do just this.

At this point you will most likely want to schedule the patient for a consultation appointment to present the treatment plan. To lead into this you might consider the following:

The success of any restorative work depends on a comprehensive diagnosis in order to be effective. And that is what I've done today. What I need to do now is take some time to study your radiographs, the findings of the clinical examination, all that we discussed, your wants and concerns and (then list anything else such as study models, etc.) and work out the most effective treatment plan for your individual needs. What I'd like to do is schedule you to return in approximately 5-7 days for a treatment plan consultation... that will give me the time necessary to give your situation every consideration. Then, we'll discuss the most effective treatment plan for you. How does that sound?

Great. Is there anything else you would like to tell me or want me to know before you leave today?

If the patient asks you how much it will cost, obviously you won't know yet because you haven't take the time to study the case and work out the treatment plan. It is best to not get into the issue of fees at this time if at all possible. In many businesses it is appropriate to ask how much a person would be willing to contribute toward the product, but in dentistry, we should be presenting the very best treatment plan for the patient, without our first concern being how much it will cost. Think about responding this way:

Mrs. Jones, I can't tell you what it will be until I complete the treat-

Mrs. Jones, I can't tell you what it will be until I complete the treatment plan. But let me ask you this: Do you have a budget for your dentistry? (Here you'll at least get an idea of what the patient is thinking and will help you to better prepare for the treatment plan presentation). If we are able to (then repeat his needs, wants and desires) and we can work out something that will work for your budget, when would you want to get started? If the patient brings up the insurance question, you might respond with something like this:

Mrs. Jones, I know you have insurance and I know you may be concerned about whether or not your insurance will cover recommended treatment. It is important for you to know that I don't diagnose dentistry on what the insurance company will pay. My concern is for your dental health. The treatment I recommend will be based on your individual needs...and what I would do in my mouth or my family's mouth in a similar situation...not on what the insurance company benefit is. I won't let any insurance carrier dictate what I diagnose or recommend to you. There is no substitute for poor quality when it comes to your dental health.

When you have completed the exam and are ready to dismiss the patient for the day and schedule the consultation appointment, you may want to ask the patient if anyone else besides him/herself will be involved in making a decision about proceeding with treatment. If someone else is involved, invite that person to be present when the treatment plan is presented. Obviously this will not always be possible, but in many cases you can eliminate the no's by making the presentation of the treatment plan to both parties making the decision.

Again, the treatment plan should be completed as soon as possible after the exam. If not the same day, and in most cases it probably won't be, it should be scheduled within the next 5-7 days at the longest. The longer the delay, the lower the possibility of acceptance. The patient's attention is on dental care and at its highest when they are in the dental chair. As soon as they leave the chair they begin to cool down. The disturbance lowers. The emotional involvement wanes. One study indicates that as soon as the patient leaves the chair, the acceptance decreases by 30%...and continues to decrease an additional 10% for every week that passes.

risen to 90%!

The Consultation Appointment

When the patient returns for the consultation appointment, you actually finish the need identification stage of the selling process. This cannot be completed in full until you do the diagnosis.

It's been a few days since the patient was in and you'll want to bring him back to the *emotional* level he was at when he left. Take him back to that *disturbance.* Now is the time for you to *acknowledge the needs of the patient* by repeating his concerns, wants and desires that were identified in the intial appointment. Recap what you understand his or her goals to be. Then, present your findings (needs) in full...and *relate them to the patients wants and desires.* Remember, you want to help the patient move from "needs" to "wants." If you have an intraoral camera, it can be used very effectively, once again, to "walk through the patients mouth" and show the patient what you are talking about as you present your findings and diagnosis. Once you have done this, an easy way to check the emotional level of the patient and gain agreement is to ask a question. Here are a couple examples:

If we can achieve all that you would like to achieve and provide all the benefits with a treatment plan that fits with your (budget, schedule, comfort requirements...whatever might be a concern), when would you want to get started?

You've indicated you want your teeth to be whiter than they are right now...isn't that correct? If we can accomplish this for you, when would you want to get started?

Mr. Jones, you've indicated to me that your most important concern is keeping your teeth your entire life...isn't that correct? If we can begin a treatment plan that will allow you to do just this, when would you want to get started?

These kinds of question really help nail down the patients level of commitment, find out if he is sold on the need, or has a strong commitment, find out if he is sold on the need, or has a strong enough desire to act. If you find hesitation here, going on with the solution (treatment plan) may prove futile.

> If you find you don't yet have the agreement
> you need to find out what the problem or
> objection is, and any other concerns of the patient.

The entire need identification step is geared toward finding out what motivates the patient, as well as completing the clinical examination so you can make your diagnosis and recommended treatment plan. Once this is completed you then direct the *needs discovered* to the *patient's motivation* during the solution stage of the selling process.

Let's once again remember how important gaining the agreement is in the entire selling process. If you reach a point where the patient does not agree, then you have virtually lost the sale right there unless you can handle the objection. By asking questions, if there is disagreement, you will know about it right away and can work on turning it around. If you don't, however, and you continue on through the rest of the process, you risk finding a big NO at the end...and you'll wonder why.

Once the clinical exam is completed, you've consulted with your patient about his needs, and you've gained agreement, it's time to move to the next stage. Remember, the patient must be disturbed before you move on. If he isn't, the likelihood of him being "moved to action" when you come to the treatment plan presentation may be marginal.

Chapter 28

STEP V: PRESENTING THE SOLUTION

The objective of the solution stage is to *present the treatment plan, sell the benefits, relieve the patient's concern* (need, want, desire) by showing how you can handle it, and *gain agreement* on your solution. The patient's attitude at this stage will be curious and disturbed. Disturbed because you've just brought him to that point as you identified the needs (and related his wants to his needs), and curious as to what you can do to solve the problem or take care of the want or desire.

> The buying decision at this point is that
> *your* treatment plan is ideal...not that *any*
> treatment plan is ideal, but that your's is.

You don't want to go through the process only to educate the patient about needs, and not make the sale. Yet, this is what many people continue to do. You are not a professional educator, only to have the patient leave your practice informed but untreated, and go to the next practice and make an "easy sale" for the dentist down the road do to the treatment.

During this consultation appointment, after you've brought him back to the emotional level he was at previously and discussed with him his needs and wants, now it's time to present the actual treatment plan recommendation. Let's look at the five factors of presenting the treatment plan...or solution stage of the selling process.

1.   *Present the treatment plan and the benefits.* Relate the treatment and the benefits back to what you identified as the patients wants and desires (hot buttons). There are actually five parts to communicate:

- Present what treatment needs to be done and benefits of that treatment
- Identify how many appointments will be needed
- Determine what will be done at each appointment
- Indicate how long each appointment will take
- Present the fee

Consider presenting the treatment plan in writing as well, and once you've gained agreement from the patient, have him sign the treatment plan as agreement of his acceptance. This way, any question from a patient "not remembering" what you said about any of the five steps will be circumvented, and a great deal of misunderstanding and hard feelings eliminated.

It is critically important to understand features versus benefits. People don't buy features; they buy benefits. Here's a brief story to illustrate the point.

The hardware salesman spent nearly ten minutes telling his customer how good his 3/4 inch drill bits were. "They're sharp, tough, long lasting and above all they don't cost much," the salesman said. To which the customer replied, "That's all just great, but I don't care about the 3/4 inch bits...all I want is a 3/4 inch hole!"

The customer is concerned about the benefits, not the features.

A *feature* is the actual physical characteristic
that exists regardless of the patient.

A *benefit* is how the feature relates to this particular patient's
needs, wants, desires, and the advantages it gives.
It answers the question, *"What does it mean for me?"*

For example: You diagnose that a patient needs a crown. This
patient already told you that he doesn't want any more appointments than necessary...and he wants dentistry that will last the longest time. Based on his concerns, you relate it this way:

*Mr. Jones, your tooth is fractured, which means (and then
explain the problem this creates). The tooth needs to be crowned,
which will (and translate the treatment into the benefit for the
patient).*

*When we spoke last week you indicated that you wanted your
dentistry completed in such a way that it will last the longest
possible. Isn't that correct? (Pause and let the patient respond)
Because of that, I'm going to suggest that we do a gold crown.
Gold is more durable and generally lasts longer than a large
silver filling. How does that sound?*

Perhaps you have a patient with an involved treatment plan. You
might approach him with:

*Mrs. Jones, we have a lot of problems to solve here. I have
approached your situation with what I believe to be the most
effective and best way to treat your dental needs. I haven't
researched your insurance and I don't know what your budget is,
but I am going to recommend to you what I would do in my
mouth...or what I would do in the mouth of my wife or best friend.*

A feature may have more than one benefit, and what may be a
benefit to one patient is not a benefit to another. Let's say two patients have quite substantial diastemas. For one, the concern has to
do with her looks. For the other, the major concern is how it affects
his speech. Even though the treatment is the same, you would discuss the treatment necessary to correct the situation, and then for
the patient concerned with looks you would say *"...and by doing
this we will create that new smile you've always wanted. And that is*

important to you, isn't it?" For the patient concerned with his speech, you could say, *"...and by doing this we will eliminate the problems of speech associated with the diastema and allow you lisp-free speaking, and that was a concern of your's, wasn't it?"*

A solution with impact is created by forming word pictures and sell-ing benefits. Most patients won't be interested so much in how the process is completed...they aren't usually interested in what it takes to do a crown or root canal...but they do care about what that crown or root canal will do for them. We must always remember that people don't buy cleanings, crowns, bridges, dentures, bleaching, or any other *procedure.* What they do buy is a prettier smile, a healthier mouth, elimination or reduction of pain, ability to chew comfortably, greater self esteem, convenience, comfort, ability to keep their teeth for a lifetime, etc. *They are buying positive experi-ences.* And that's what you must communicate to them. It's impor-tant to make the connection for patients between what you have to offer and what they want.

One poll taken recently indicates that Americans have conflicting ideas concerning periodontal disease. Of the 1,000 respondents, 80% be-lieved they did not have periodontal disease...yet 70% reported having experienced at least one of the following: bleeding gums; swollen, painful or receding gums; a change in bite; or loose teeth.

Further, only 36% of the adults surveyed who had bleeding gums indicated they had told their dentist about the problem. And only 30% of those who have experienced warning signs of gum disease are worried about developing periodontal problems down the road. The shocking fact is that 41% of these respondents said that losing their teeth was one of their biggest fears concerning their oral health!

It is also important not to prejudge or try to determine in ad-vance what a patient will accept or reject. It is our moral and ethi-cal responsibility to give the patient every opportunity to choose what is the very best for him or herself. If the patient has already indicated to you somewhere along the way that money is a prob-lem, you might lead in with something such as:

Mrs. Jones, I'm in a bit of a quandary here because you told me previously that you have limited funds for your dental treatment. I have studied your situation over and over, looking at every conceivable approach, and in order to save your teeth (or restore your teeth to optimal health...or accomplish what you've told me you want to accomplish) there is no way I can do it optimally any other way. This may not be workable for you, but I can't make that decision for you. What I'd like to do is present my findings and treatment plan to you, and we'll take discuss it from there.

Call reluctance in sales is something a great percentage of sales-people are plagued with. In dentistry, one area of call reluctance is in presenting the very best treatment plan to a patient. It has been estimated that 94% of all dentists have call reluctance. That is the reason dentists don't present comprehensive treatment plans...they fear rejection, that the treatment plan won't be accepted.

A professional colleague of mine who lives about 150 miles from Portland has been seeing one dentist in his hometown for a number of years. When he met Norm after we were married, and got to know him, he began wondering about the kind of treatment he was getting from his dentist. Finally he made the decision to fly over and have Norm do a new patient exam, followed by a treatment plan and consultation appointment a week or so later. When Norm did the new patient exam he found major work needing to be done.

During the consultation Norm presented the findings and the treatment plan based on what he would want in his mouth...or what he would recommend in my mouth in a similar situation.

A month or so after the consultation and a couple appointments later I met with this friend for coffee when he was in town. He said to me, "You know, Cheryl, what I really appreciated about Norm is not just how congenial he is, or how great the team is...but that he was up front and open with me and told me like it is. I've felt for a long time that my previous dentist was just patching problems when they couldn't be put off any longer. I don't feel as though he ever really told me what was really go-

ing on in my mouth. Of course, I wasn't sure, but I felt it. It feels so good to know that Norm has done a thorough exam and diagnosis and now I'll really get the best treatment possible."

When you present your treatment plan, whatever it is, *if you truly believe it is the very best for the patient,* that is most likely what the patient will accept. If you don't really believe it, and have presented a treatment option based on the patient's insurance benefits or what you *assume* the patient can afford, the patient will pick up on that and in many situations no amount of selling will get you the order.

2. Get the patient involved. Appeal to all the patient's senses, once again, both emotionally and logically. Vividly create the mental picture. As you are going through the findings, state what the situation is with each tooth and then use two key words, **left untreated,** and then go into what the consequences are of doing nothing. Create a vivid picture in the patient's mind.

3. Emphasize value. People are cost conscious today and value is important in order to justify the fee. Here it is extremely important to understand that you must convince yourself first.

> If you don't believe the value the patient will
> receive is equal to or greater than your fee...
> then you won't be able to hide your doubt.

When this is the case, the patient will pick up on what you are trying *not* to communicate, and you'll be on the receiving end of an objection you cannot handle effectively. When value is high, resistance is low.

4. Be prepared to offer validation. Validation is the support for the patient to feel good about agreeing to the solution and feeling comfortable this is a necessary, safe, and effective procedure. Guarantees are great, where appropriate. Demonstrations, literature, and third party influence is also validation. If you have a past case that is particularly appropriate, relate that.

5. Get patient feedback . All the way through, gain agreement with each feature and benefit you relate.

> *Mr. Jones, you indicated your concerns about your overall dental health, and that you wanted to do everything possible to keep your teeth for your lifetime. Isn't that correct?*

> *After taking a few hours to study your dental situation, I have come up with a treatment plan that, once completed, if you do what is necessary on a homecare basis and you come in regularly every six months so we can do our part (or whatever intervals are appropriate), this should put you into a position for strong dental health. Does this sound like it would meet your objectives?*

You want all the feedback from the patient you can get. You need to know, with every step of the treatment plan presentation, that the patient is still with you and is in agreement. This feedback gives you clues as to the patient's readiness for making a commitment. Use phrases such as, "...and this is important to you, isn't it?" or "...and this is your greatest concern, isn't it?"

Power Phrases in the Solution

Are you familiar with power phrases? Power phrases can be used throughout the selling process, but they are particularly effective in the solution, in helping create word pictures, and in the close. Early in my own selling career it was impressed upon me that an effective presentation was essential, and that it isn't so much *what* you say as *how* you say it. Power phrases are excellent tools to get attention, to keep attention from wandering, and to maintain interest. They are also great in the close! Every word in a power phrase is carefully placed for greatest impact. The meaning of a power phrase might be communicated in several different ways using many different words, but when communicated as a power phrase the meaning gets through dramatically. Here are a few examples of general power phrases:

Your salary increase will become effective when you do.

A label on a box full of fish in a Seattle post office read: If not delivered within five days, don't bother.

You can't solve a permanent problem with a temporary solution.

Your people are the greatest asset on your balance sheet. Isn't it a good idea to invest in that asset?

Life insurance costs less to buy than not to buy.

Here's an example you could use in your practice:

Mrs. Smith, you have the beginning of...........but if we take care of it now, at your stage it can be completely reversed. There is nothing to be alarmed about yet...but there is if it is left untreated.

Before we move on, let's capsulize the solution. Recap the problem and needs, and present the treatment plan by relating the treatment and the benefits back to the patient's individual needs, wants and desires. Gain agreement that the treatment needs to be done, and that the patient wants you to do the dentistry...not just any dentist. Be sure to offer the advantages of completing treatment and include the words "left untreated" and then go into the possible consequences if the treatment is put off.

Help the Patient Buy

Many people need the reassurance that the decisions they make are okay decisions. This is true also in dentistry. Help your patients feel they deserve the benefits of the treatment. If they don't believe it, they often won't buy it *even when they could easily afford it!*

Sometimes we don't present the whole picture because we prejudge their financial situation and don't feel comfortable presenting the full treatment plan and verbalizing the investment needing to be made (the fee!). Step back just a moment and look at it from a different perspective. If you don't tell your patients the whole story, each time they come to you you must tell them another crown (or other treatment) needs to be done (because their mouth is falling apart piece by piece). They will begin to lose confidence: it seems you're always looking for more dentistry to do. Credibility can be lost as the question marks in their mind arise.

On the other hand, when you do a comprehensive exam with full diagnosis and corresponding treatment plan, you are presenting your patient with the very best you have to offer. You can see the completed picture and it looks good. You feel good about it. It's the kind of dentistry you spent all those years in dental school and continuing education to learn. The one-at-a-time approach is the bandaid approach. Not only will the patient begin to lose confidence and question your motives and the way you work, but the opportunity for an even worse situation to develop is magnified and could compromise what would otherwise be a great outcome.

> Diagnose and present a treatment plan so all your
> patients have the opportunity to have a beautiful smile
> and a healthy mouth with the best possible function.
> Give them the opportunity to have the
> very best dentistry possible.

And remember, proper treatment planning involves not only making the diagnosis and communicating that to the patient, but it also involves *writing out* (1) what needs to be done, (2) the number of appointments the patient will need to complete the treatment, (3) what will be done at each appointment, (4) how long each appointment will take, and (5) what the fees will be.

Think about your patients right now. Individually. Can you say that the majority of your patients have the very best dentistry you know how to do in their mouths? If not, why not? Is it really because of money, or time, or fear? Or is it because you did not offer...and learn to sell...the very best dental treatment plan possible?

Chapter 29

STEP VI: CLOSING

People often have erroneous ideas of closing the sale...in fact,
entirely *too much emphasis* is placed on closing. Closing is not some
magic moment in the selling process; it is a natural progression of
the presentation. Closing is simply implementing the agreed upon
solution. With the *needs* determined and presented, and the *solution* mutually agreed upon, commitment to implementing the solution is natural.

On the other hand, *not enough emphasis* is placed here. I say
that because so many people in selling, including dentistry, don't
close! They simply let the patient off the hook. They present the
treatment plan, then say something like "Well, do you have any
questions?" And when the patient doesn't have any, or even if he
does, the next common response from the dentist is, "Well, why
don't you think about it and give our receptionist a call when you've
had the time to consider what we've just discussed."

Selling dentistry is like any other product or service in one
respect...the longer the time between the presentation of the product or service (treatment plan presentation) and the patient's deci-

sion to go ahead with treatment, the less likely the patient is to purchase.

> The acceptance rate for treatment drops substantially
> as soon as the patient walks out your door.

If you haven't scheduled the treatment, the likelihood is good that the patient will not act on the treatment until some time in the future when an emergency occurs or pain intrudes...when they are disturbed!

We have allowed insurance companies to be a factor here because many of us have believed for so long (and many still do) that predeterminations were necessary. The real situation is that predeterminations most often are not only *not required*, but they are *nonbinding*. They do not guarantee payment. They simply determine eligibility on the date of predetermination, and guarantee nothing when the actual treatment is completed.

One report indicates that according to dental insurance company statistics 40% of dental patients will forego treatment if it is delayed by just three weeks from the date of diagnosis. Some industry figures estimate the amount of dentistry lost due to the time lag between patient diagnosis, treatment plan acceptance, and the 30 day or more wait for predeterminations to be returned to be in the high 70% range. Whatever the actual figure might be, it is a remarkable loss...for your patient and for you. Rather than send in a predetermination next time, have your staff call the insurance company and ask this question, *"According to the contract, will you refuse payment to an otherwise eligible patient if no predetermination was completed?"*

As we move into the close, the attitude of the patient may be a little cooled off as you approach the question. However, if you have followed the process as presented, the patient should be eager to "take the dentistry home" so to speak. It's time for the close.

> The buying decision to be made is that
> now is the time to buy.
> Your objective in this stage of the sales process
> is to ask for the sale...to ask the patient to accept
> the treatment plan and schedule the treatment.

The most important part of the sales process is you...and you need to remember the ABC's of closing...Always Be Closing! That means gaining agreement at every step along the way. When you have done that, the actual closing part of the process, asking for the patient to accept the treatment plan and schedule treatment, is a logical conclusion to the rest of the presentation. If they have agreed all along, it is natural to believe they are with you, believe in what you have suggested, and will take the scheduling steps.

Closing begins way back in the approach and it is sparked by your attitude, appearance, what you say and how you say it...as well as by your team's attitude, appearance, what they say and how they say it. It continues throughout the entire time you are working with the patient as you gain agreement at every successive stage. In fact, your close is well under way with the patient's first yes or nod of agreement, when they first walk in the door!

We learned to ask questions earlier, and as the patient continually agrees it is increasingly difficult not to continue to agree. Closing really does begin at the beginning! If you follow the Principled Selling process step by step, gaining agreement at every stage, the final decision comes as a natural part of the sequence.

Selling is like putting on a glove one finger at a time. First you take the measurement of the hand to determine what size glove will fit (need identification). After you determine which glove is best suited, you present the solution, explaining why this glove is the ideal glove for the customer (features and benefits based on their needs, wants, desires). With each yes throughout the presentation the glove goes on a little further. By the time you have completed the solution, the glove is all the way on and it fits perfectly. Now comes the close. For the patient to say no now means he has to reverse the process and *take off the glove that has become his*...and that is harder than leaving it on! It fits...it is already his. And that's how your entire presentation with your patient must be. By the time you are ready to ask the closing question the patient should already feel that the dentistry you are recommending belongs to him.

As you present the solution and come to the close, be sure you always emphasize value. Emphasize the service provided the patient, the benefits the patient will gain, and don't place the emphasis on the fee. Your acceptance will increase when you do.

If you find resistance in patients accepting treatment, go back and review the steps leading to the close to see where you skipped a step or were ineffective. Remember, if you do not have a *qualified* prospect (prospective patient) you will not be able to close the sale no matter how hard you try.

Asking the Closing Question

There are many ways to ask the closing questions. Let's identify a few here that can be used in your practice.

*The first is the **alternative or choice close.*** This is a question with two answers. Either answer confirms the patient's decision to accept treatment.

> *Would you prefer to schedule your first appointment this week, or would next week be better? (Not...When would you like to get started?)*

> *Would you like to handle this with your Visa or Master card, or will you be paying by check? (Not...Would you like to pay for this by check?)*

> *Do you prefer treatment plan A or treatment plan B? (Obviously used only where there is an alternate treatment plan.)*

Notice that none of these three questions can be answered with a yes or no. If you simply asked, "Would you prefer to schedule your first appointment this week?"you leave yourself open for a "no" response, which means you then have to ask another question. Give your patient a choice from the start...and when he answers one of the choices, you have made the sale! Also be aware that most people tend to take the second choice offered in an alternate close situation. Therefore, position your preferred option last.

*The second type of closing is the **obvious close.*** Read carefully: The person who asks the last question is in control. Many, many sales have been lost because the salesperson wasn't really hearing a prospect and the prospect asked a question to which the salesperson replied "Yes," "No," or "Of course." For example, "Can I get it done before my reunion the fifteenth of next month? Some dentists would answer, "Sure" and drop it at that. Then they must ask another question to find out if the patient is ready to schedule. Instead, when a question like this is asked, respond with"Would you like to have it done before your reunion?" When the patient answers "yes" you can move right into scheduling.

Although there are many different types of closing, the alternative or choice close, and the obvious close, are among the easiest to use and the least aggressive.

The Ben Franklin close is one that may be useful in situations where a person is indecisive. When presented correctly it can be very effective. You are at the closing question, but the patient is having a difficult time making up his or her mind. Simply draw a "T" on a pad of paper and label one side "pluses" and one side "minuses." Then put a few numbers down the plus side (say one through five) and put only one or two on the minus side. Then say to the patient,

> *Mrs. Jones, it seems like you are having a difficult time making*
> *this decision. Why don't we do this very simply by listing all*
> *the pluses and all the minuses and see which side weighs heaviest.*
> *Okay, here's the pencil...it's your decision, so write them down in*
> *your words.*

Then, as you are working on the plus side, help the patient remember all the things she agreed to or liked...all the benefits of having the treatment. When you get to the negative side, let the patient come up with these herself. By the time you are completed, the patient will have her own balance sheet and should be able to make the decision more easily.

The *simply ask close* is to simply ask the question in a straight forward manner. "Mrs. Jones, when would you like to get started with your treatment," or "Mrs. Jones, where do we go from here?" or "How does this sound?"Caution here, however. This seems almost too easy and unless you have really done your job well in *every step of the selling process* this close won't work, at least not successfully. But, when you know you have completed all steps of the Principled Selling process in order and have fully gained agreement, then you can feel sure you are in a position to ask this type of low key closing question.

When it comes to closing, remember that it is your belief that will greatly affect the outcome of your treatment plan presentation. It requires *conviction*...conviction that what you are presenting is what is truly best for the patient, and conviction that the service you are providing is equal to or greater than the fee required. Without this belief, this conviction, everyone loses.

The C in Close stands for Conviction.
When you remove the C all you have left is lose!

And finally, remember that once the patient leaves your office without accepting the treatment plan and scheduling the first appointment, the likelihood of the patient ever scheduling this treatment begins to diminish rapidly.

When you've completed the process properly and the patient has become "thirsty," and you've gained agreement all along the way, then you'll know where your patient stands long before you ask the closing question.

It is important to help your patient with options financially and help them to be able to have the treatment. Often people don't even know they really want something until they see it really is a possibility to have it. If they feel there is no way, they'll even talk themselves into believing they can do without it.

Needs, dreams, and desires are sometimes
shaped by what a person believes is possible.

If the patient hesitates or is unsure and says, " I don't know. I'm not sure." Follow up with a question to get to the bottom of his thinking.

Mr. Jones. I guess I don't understand. You've indicated to me that you want (and again capsulize his expressed needs, wants, desires)...and we've discussed how your situation of (then describe what his condition is and how without treatment he will not be able to achieve his need, want, desire). You've also indicated that you are truly concerned about the consequences if this condition is left untreated. I'm not sure what it is that you're hesitating about. Can you help me out with this? Do you have any other concerns we haven't discussed?

Closing is not just the *final* part of making the sale. It is a part of the entire process all the way up to the final decision. It begins with the approach and continues throughout your presentation culminating in the closing question. When you've followed the process completely and thoroughly...selling is fun...and it is profitable....*and every person involved wins!*

Chapter 30

STEP VII: REFERRALS

The seventh step of the Principled Selling process is asking for referrals. When you and your team don't ask for referrals you make continual building of the practice more difficult than necessary. It is important to develop the habit of asking for referrals regularly, often, and at every opportunity.

Obtaining referrals is the most effective form of marketing. But if it is so effective why don't people consistently ask for referrals? Probably because they don't really understand how effective it can be; they don't understand that people really do want to help; or they don't feel confident because they don't know what to say or how to ask. Just as it is important to know ahead of time what you are going to say in the other steps of the Principled Selling process, it is important for you to learn to ask for referrals. When you know how you will ask, you will be much more confident in asking; when you are confident in asking, you will be much less likely to "forget" to ask.

Several times I've been in an office and overhead a patient ask a team member, "Does doctor see any new patients?" or some similar question. The response is, "Yes" and nothing more is said. This is like winning the lottery and never going to pick-up the money, or winning a vacation to Hawaii but never taking it! We need to listen for these openings for referrals, and then maximize the opportunity.

> No matter how much a person likes you and your practice,
> if they don't feel comfortable referring to you...they won't.
> They need to know that your doors are open for referrals,
> and that you welcome them openly.

If you've done your best and the patient has had a good experience in your practice, then asking for referrals should come easily. After all, the patient has just been helped tremendously. He or she is feeling good, the pain is relieved, perhaps a positive result has just been experienced with a cosmetic issue, or a problem has been solved. Whatever the situation, the patient is pleased and feels good about you and your practice. Your part is to ask the question, and the patient will most likely want to help you out with referrals. What you want to communicate to your patient is that if they really like their experience with you, to tell a friend (but if they don't, to tell you).

> When you take care of your patients,
> they will take care of you.

Perhaps you're getting pretty good results in the referrals category, but if you're only asking periodically (or not asking at all) can you imagine what your results might be if you really had a "system" for obtaining referrals? The best patients you will ever have are those referred by your best patients. And it costs virtually nothing!

During your morning huddle, determine which patients you will ask for referrals today. Identify who meets your preferred patient profile, and then divide the names among yourself and the other staff members as to who will be responsible for asking so not all ask the same person. Don't leave it to chance. As you practice this and it becomes habit, each team member will become stronger and feel comfortable asking, and as it becomes habit you will naturally move into the referral process regularly. When you do, you'll see your new patient flow increase substantially.

Mr. Smith, you are one of my favorite patients. You always keep your appointments and arrive on time. We really appreciate that. And you're always so friendly and cooperative. In our experience, our very best patients are referred by our very best patients...and that's how we feel about you. We would welcome any referral of friends or family or co-workers that you would like to send us. We'd love to have more patients like you.

Usually the referral question is best asked when the patient is fresh and interested, rather than at the end of the appointment, although there are no hard and fast rules. The ideal is to obtain specific names of people your patients want to refer. Rather than say something like, "Mr. Smith, we really enjoy having you in our practice and we would consider it a compliment if you would refer other people like yourself to us," say:

"Mr. Smith, I'll bet you're really enthusiastic about seeing the final result today, aren't you? What does your wife (family, girlfriend, significant other) think? Have you told anyone where you work?" This is a great question to be asked by the assistant or hygienist.

Depending upon the answer, if someone has shown an interest, ask, "Is there anyone who has expressed an interest in having some changes made in (the appearance of their smile, the color of their teeth, etc)?" If the patient answers yes, respond, "Great, would you feel comfortable sharing their name with us so we could give them a call and introduce ourselves?"

If asking for a specific name does not feel appropriate, then continue with, "Mr. Smith, here's my business card. Would you be kind enough to tell (interested party's name) about us and give her our card. Ask her to call and let her know that we will take special care of her."

Another way to handle this is to ask the referrer how you could contact that person and then either send a letter of introduction and then call, or simply make the call.

Ms. White, my name is _____ from Dr. _____'s dental office. Mr. Smith, a patient of ours and as we understand a (friend, co-worker, etc.) of yours mentioned to us that you expressed an interest in (state what was of interest). We'd like to introduce ourselves to you and let you know that we would be happy to be of service if you are looking for a new dentist or have a particular concern at this time.

As the patient leaves and is walked to the front desk, make mention to the receptionist with Mr. Smith present, "(Referral's name) may be calling because she is interested in (bleaching). Mr. Smith is going to tell her about our office." This cements in the patient's mind the importance of this referral and the value you place on it.

Another option for obtaining referrals is to have a referral card printed that says something like this:

Dr. (your name), I am so pleased with my experience in your dental office and the care from you and your entire team that I am referring_____.

Please give _____ the same attention and care that you give me.

Sincerely,

Then you can present a referral card or two to the patient you would like to approach for referrals with this:

Mrs. Jones, may I ask a favor from you? Here are two patient referral cards. I'd really appreciate it if you would give them to two of your friends, family or co-workers you believe would appreciate the same kind of attention and care you have received in our practice. Just fill in their names on the two appropriate lines and sign your name so I can be sure to thank you when they come in.

Throughout your day, in addition to the specific individuals identified in the huddle to approach for referrals, always be listening and looking for ways to tie in a referral. Pick up on what the patient says, whether it is a compliment or anything else that is appropriate. Here are some common openings:

Patient says to the assistant:	"Gee, Dr. _____ is really gentle."
Patient says to the hygienist:	"My teeth have never felt so clean, they really feel great."
Patient says to receptionist:	"This is really a nice office, I'm glad we decided to come here."
Or others such as:	"Are you taking new patients?" "I've never had such a complete exam before. Do all dentists do this? "Wow, that was great! I didn't even feel it!"

All these questions and statements are openings to ask for referrals on the spot. Here are a few examples of how you and your staff might respond.

Thank you, Mr. _____. It's very important to us to be as gentle as we can with our patients and we're glad you feel this way. If you know of anyone looking for a dental practice with our care and concern, we'd really appreciate you telling them about us.

We're glad you decided to come here, too, and we're pleased that you are happy with your dental experience here. We'd be delighted if you would mention us to anyone you know who might be looking for a (family dentist, general dentist, orthodontist or whatever your specialty). We'd be pleased to welcome them to our practice.

You're absolutely right. This is a very complete exam. This is an essential part of being able to provide you with the very best dental care possible. And no, not every dentist provides this comprehensive exam. If you know of anyone who is interested in the very best dental care possible, we'd feel privileged if you would tell them about us. (Or, "Do you know of anyone who is interested in having the very best dental care possible?")

It is important to understand that most people will refer people who are similar to themselves. If you have a patient with mega-financial problems and it is difficult to obtain payment for their services, it is likely that referrals from this person would have similar problems. On the other hand, if you have a patient with whom you communicate easily and get along well, and who is in a good financial position, it's highly likely that referrals from this person will be much like your patient. Therefore, *target your best patients for referrals.* People who keep their appointments, who cooperate with you, those with whom you've had the great successes, who have had major work, who have just finished something they feel really great about, are all people who could easily be approached for referrals.

Don't wait until you complete all the work on a patient before you ask for referrals. Once you have built a relationship and confidence in that relationship, the new patient's confidence in you is high. While enthusiasm is high, ask for referrals. One further comment here. Although it is helpful to have every team member involved in the referral process, surveys do indicate that a higher referral rate is achieved when the doctor does the asking.

Another indirect way of asking for referrals is to have a sign in the office that lets patients know you welcome referrals.

Once you receive a referral from a patient, be sure to thank the referrer. A hand-written letter or note from you (or from the entire team with all their signatures) is well received. It can be as simple as "Thank you for your confidence in us by referring Ms. White." Or, "Thank you for referring Ms. White. We appreciate your confidence." The best time to send the thank you note is the day the referred patient schedules his or her appointment. That way even if the patient doesn't actually show up on the appointed day you won't forget to thank the referral. Also, if the new patient didn't show up (or was thinking about not showing up) the referring patient might be talking with that prospective patient and encourage him or her to go in, or to call and reschedule if it is after the fact.

If you receive several referrals from one person you might want to consider something more such as flowers, tickets to a sporting or cultural event in your community, a certificate for dinner for two or anything else you feel is appropriate. Experiences of gratitude and thanks are rare and are therefore long remembered. People like to know their efforts are appreciated. When they are, they will do all they can to help you even more the next time around. Remember the principle: What gets rewarded generally gets repeated.

If you've got a great team, a great practice, and you know your patients are dedicated and loyal to you, yet you find even when you ask for referrals that you are unproductive, take a look around. Are there problems in your practice you haven't identified? Maybe there are some things your patients have learned to live with and have developed a certain comfort level with you, but they haven't referred others to your practice because they feel embarrassed, and are not comfortable in making the referral. How does your office look? Is it neat, clean, up-to-date? Does it look like it would be "safe"? What about your equipment? Is it up-to-date? Does your team communicate that they like working there, that they like each other, that you have good relationships? Do you and your team members refrain from discussing personal problems with patients?

And finally, consider this. Asking for referrals is a part of the Principled Selling process. *If you forget to ask, or for whatever other reason don't ask, you have not completed the selling process.* When you implement a regular referral system in your practice, you will find that you can increase your new patient flow tremendously. The people who are pleased, enthusiastic, and fully satisfied with the care they receive from you will be your voluntary cheerleaders...they just need to know that you'd like them to be.

Chapter 31

STEP VIII: CRITIQUE

The reason you are in dentistry is to help other people, to provide a good income for yourself and your family, to provide you the freedom that being in business for yourself can give, and to allow you options. Right? And the reason you study, attend seminars or study clubs, and read is to gain further knowledge to ensure your success in dentistry, and to keep up with the latest. Isn't that right? It is only natural then, that you will want to increase your effectiveness and closing ratio as you go along. Doing this means you work smarter, not harder. Critiquing your presentation will help you to continually make progress.

Think through the process with each patient. How did you do? What did you do that was very good? What seemed to really capture the attention and interest of your patient? Then try doing more of it in the future. Did you notice that something didn't go well or smoothly? Where did you feel you "lost" the patient, or felt you were out of control of the process? Identify these, go back and review the basics and determine how you will avoid that situation or do better the next time. If you felt really great about the entire presentation, identify why. Or, if you didn't gain agreement to move ahead with the treatment plan, try to identify why not. Success would be meaningless if there was no opportunity for failure. Not even the most outstanding salesperson makes every sale. If we can learn to analyze the sales we don't make, as well as those we do make, we can make our failures, and our successes, work for us. Here are a few questions to help you begin the process of critiquing yourself:

Did you have a patient who was a "qualified prospect?"
How much did you get to know about your patient?
Did you identify the patient's hot buttons....wants, desires?
How was your patient greeted by each person on your team (including you)?
What about the your appearance, and the appearance of your team members?
What about the appearance of the office?
Did you provide outstanding service?
Did the patient feel he/she was cared for?
Did you give the patient your undivided attention?
Did you refrain from arguing when objections were expressed by the patient?
Did you inspire confidence by sincere enthusiasm, eye contact, and body language?
Were there other decision makers who should have been involved?
Did you allow yourself sufficient time for each part of the process?
Did you have a well thought out and written treatment plan to present to the patient?
Were you able to relate the treatment needed back to the patient's wants and desires?
Did the patient become "thirsty" for what needed to be done?
Were you able to handle objections effectively?
Did you speak in terms the patient could understand?
Were you enthusiastic throughout your involvement with the patient?
Did you really listen to your patient?
Did you uncover any hidden objections?

Did you go too fast?

Did you gain agreement on each point before going on to the next?

Did you ask enough questions to clearly identify what is important to the patient?

Did you drown the patient in a sea of facts that he or she was unable to absorb or understand?

Did you ask the patient to accept the treatment plan?

Professional salespeople are continually looking for ways to improve. The salespeople who are less professional often repeat their first year in the business over and over. In fact, some people who have been in selling (or any business for that matter) for 15 years really don't have 15 years experience. They have one year's experience fifteen times over. There is a difference!

Invest the time both by yourself and with your team to critique how you are doing and make the necessary adjustments.

Chapter 32

STEP VIX: SERVICE

The ninth step in the Principled Selling process is service. There is a saying in sales that the salesperson's job doesn't end when he sees the taillights of his customer's car. In fact, it is just beginning. The same is true in dentistry. We want to develop a patient clientele...that means patients who return over and over again, and who feel good about and will make referrals to the practice. If we don't service our patients, however, they just might go somewhere else.

Providing quality service means building good will. The U.S. Supreme Court defines Good Will as *the inclination of a buyer to return to the source of his/her satisfaction.* And that's what service is all about for you, getting your patients to return over and over again, and to refer others to your practice as well.

Recognize clearly that you are *selling* in dentistry. Not only are you selling your product (the actual dentistry to be done) but you are selling your service (the care and assistance your patient receives at every step along the way). The biggest difference you have between your practice and the practice down the road is you....and each and every member of your team. What is it you provide that they don't and can't get somewhere else?

Just the other day I was in Norm's office to conduct a staff meeting. I was standing by the front desk when the last patient, who had just had a crown seated, was leaving. Here's the scenario:

Two weeks prior, Norm had been covering for another dentist who was out of town on a ten day vacation. During that time a patient of this doctor had called with a fractured tooth. The patient needed a crown, which Norm proceeded to do since the other doctor would not return for several days.

When the patient arrived in our office to have the crown seated the day of our staff meeting, he told our receptionist he had just come from the hospital where his dad was having open heart surgery and that he would be returning there just as soon as he left our office. Our assistant, Linda, and Norm were informed of this situation by our receptionist.

When Linda took the patient back to seat him she said, "I understand your father is having open heart surgery at this moment. I'll say a prayer for him." Then, as the patient was having the crown seated Linda was doing her usual omforting with her small pats on the shoulder of the patient. Norm, too, told the patient that he would keep his dad in his prayers.

Finally, with treatment completed the patient returned to the front desk to pay. I was standing there and said, "We'll keep your Dad in our prayers. Thank you for coming in, it was a pleasure to serve you."

As the patient walked across the reception room floor and reached the door, he put his hand on the door knob, turned around to face us and said, shaking his head, "I can't believe it. I can't believe the service here. I've never experienced anything like this in a medical or dental office. It almost makes it worth it to break a tooth just to come in!"

That's what service does. And this wasn't even our patient!

Service doesn't just involve the clinical part of dentistry. It is how each of the team members greet and treat the patient. It is how the financial matters are handled. Are there options for your patients when it comes to payment? Are your patients greeted with a smile and friendliness that lets them know they are truly welcome in your practice, that you are glad they are there? Do you focus the conversation on your patients? Do they feel listened to and cared for? These are all parts of service while the patient is in your practice.

But what about the service beyond? Here are some questions to ask yourself relating to service.

Do you call your patients after an involved procedure to see how they are doing?

Do you let them know you really care?

Do you treat your patients as well as you would treat a guest in your home?

Do you return phone calls to a concerned patient or a patient with a question as quickly as possible?

Do you follow-up when a patient has not scheduled the treatment needing to be done?

Do you let your patients know when it is time to return for their hygiene appointments if they didn't schedule before they left your office at the previous appointment?

Do you send a thank you to new patients for selecting your practice?

Do you send a thank you to every person who refers a patient?

If a patient tells you they are taking a vacation, do you make a note about it in the chart and ask them about it the next time they are in?

Do you send a congratulations card when you hear or read of something notable a patient has done?

Do you send a congratulations card when you know a patient has had a baby?

Do you send a wedding card when you know a patient is getting married?

Or a sympathy card when a patient has lost a loved one?

Or a get well card when a patient has had to cancel because of illness?

Are all staff members friendly, positive, responsible, prompt, tactful, thoughtful, understanding, and sincere?

In other words, do you go the extra mile? The extra time and the little cost involved will take you miles and miles in building your practice.

Service also involves handling the negative situations or complaints that arise, and handling them quickly and efficiently. Complaints are a normal part of every business, regardless of the industry, and they offer you the opportunity to show your patients why you really are the best practice for their dental care. If you handle complaints and problems properly, they will actually help you solidify the relationship and build trust. The service question to ask here is:

Do you handle complaints or problems as they arise, rather than ducking them or trying to pass them off to someone else?

Your patients are individuals who need and deserve to be cared for, treated well, and loved. They are also long term investments in your practice. It is not enough to do the dentistry and then forget the service or follow-up. Even when you have problems they should be handled in such a manner that the patient really does enjoy the experience of being in your practice. When you handle what could be negative situations directly, quickly and effectively, the patient will not only be grateful for your help, but they will be even more sold on your practice because they now know they can count on you, even when the going is tough. Following the successful handling of one of these problem situations can often be a great time to ask for referrals. The patient is happy because you resolved the issue and perhaps even verbally tells you that. Turn right around and say something like:

Thank you for your patience in working with me to get this resolved. It's great working with you Mrs. Jones and I would like to remind you,too, that we'd consider it a privilege to serve anyone you might refer to our practice. Make sure they mention your name when they call so we can be sure to thank you for the referral.

During my years in life insurance sales I told my clients when I delivered a policy that this was not the end, but the beginning of my service to them. I would say:

I took on a responsibility when you purchased this policy(ies) and I want to fulfill that responsibility as we continue working together in the years ahead. And, by my actions, concern and service, I hope to deserve the confidence you have placed in me.

Service and follow-up are often the major differences between a good dental practice and a great dental practice.

An important point of discussion as we consider service and good will is recognizing that a practice with a good reputation for dentistry and service can be torn down by an employee failing to live up to the standards of the practice that all other employees live out. It is vitally important that every team member understand and exemplify the standards of service and care with which you want be identified. One person, and all it takes is one, can cause a patient to go elsewhere looking for a new dental relationship. On the other hand, the practice that has not had the experience of being known for quality service can be brought to that level when the entire team is offering the service that is necessary for building good will.

You are in a most dynamic and rewarding profession. When it comes to how your patients perceive you and your team, and how they think about your practice (and whether or not they return), it is definitely up to you. Be good to your patients. Really care about them and they will believe in you. And when they do, they will return again and again. As you consider the service you provide your patients, think about these few words by an unknown author:

> The average man's complacent
> When he does his best to score...
> But the champion does his best...
> and then...he does a little more.

Remember: Going the extra mile is a privilege...not an obligation! Pay attention to detail, to all those moments of truth in your practice with every patient. Give your patients more than they expect in the treatment you provide, by your attitude, your concern, and your expressed interest. Consider the intangibles (the atmosphere you and your team create), as well as the tangibles.

Chapter 33

HANDLING OBJECTIONS

One word that often raises fear in the hearts and minds of inse-
cure or new salespeople is objections. Actually, objections should
be welcomed. They show us signs of interest or teach us where we
have yet to establish something with the patient. If we don't learn
how to handle objections we will miss providing dental services to
many people who are truly in need.

It is important to distinguish between objections and conditions.

Objection: **A statement by a patient indicating that he
wants/needs to know more. It is a reason for not
buying which arises because of:**

A patient's *misunderstanding* (usually based on
insufficient information or wrong information).
*A patient believes that you don't have nitrous oxide
available and the patient will not have dental work done
without it (you didn't previously have it available, but
you do now).*

A *drawback* of the product or service that exists when unable to directly satisfy the patient's dislike or dissatisfaction.
The patient prefers to be seen by someone who is very close to his home or business. You came highly recommended but you are 15 miles from either.

A patient's *lack of sufficient information.*
The patient thinks he has to pay the entire treatment plan of $6,000 up front before treatment is begun. He has not yet been informed that there are several financial options).

Condition: **A reason for not buying that actually exists. Something is missing that keeps the person from being a *qualified* prospective patient.**

The patient belongs to a dental maintenance organization and can only see doctors listed under this program, and you are not a participating doctor. *Note, however...this could still be an objection. The patient can see you if he wants to pay the cost of treatment himself.*

The patient has a need for oral surgery...and you don't do oral surgery.

The patient absolutely has no money to pay for any treatment and has no insurance. *This indicates the patient is not a qualified prospect...one of the four requirements is missing...and unless you are willing to do free dentistry on this patient you do not have a prospective patient.*

There are two times to respond to objections. They are *before they occur* and *as they occur.* The very best way to handle an objection is before it occurs. If you find that you are receiving the same objection over and over with a number of your patients, answer it before it comes up by building the response in to your presentation. By handling the objection before it is brought up by the patient as a negative, you actually turn it into a positive in the patient's mind. And when you clear the objection you clear a roadblock to the patient's acceptance of the treatment plan.

Second, handle the objection as it occurs. Perhaps the patient doesn't understand or has a misconception based on inadequate information, wrong information, or because of a previously bad experience. In this case, listen carefully to what the patient is saying. Forget about yourself and what you are going to say next and hear him out. Once you have, then tap into your knowledge reservoir of dentistry and patient relations and answer it honestly. Remember patients don't care how much you know until they know how much you care!

Some people will tell you there is a third time to answer objections: Never. This can be a mistake and a note of caution needs to be expressed. The objection may seem irrelevant or frivolous to you, but if the patient raises it more than once, you can be sure it is of concern and important to him. If this occurs you had better handle it then as your patient will think you are either ignoring him, really are not concerned about his needs, or that you have no interest in him...only in adding to your production total.

When the Patient Raises an Objection Due to a Misunderstanding

1.   Hear it out. Listen and don't interrupt.

2.   Feed it back...repeating or rephrasing the objection (to show understanding)

     In other words, you would like to *(have the treatment done, do only that part which insurance will cover, wait until the first of the year when you have new benefits established)* but you feel *(you can't afford it; you need to have insurance cover it; you need to wait until January 1; you don't deserve it)*.

3. Question it and find out what is behind the objection (especially if it is due to a drawback or misunderstanding you can't identify).

    May I ask what causes you to feel that way, Mr. Patient?

    Mrs. Patient, you must have a good reason for feeling that way...would you be kind enough to share that with me (or...mind telling me what it is)?

    Before I answer, I want to make sure I understand exactly what you mean. Will you give me some background on what it is you're concerned about?

4. Answer it. If appropriate, concede before answering (this gives the patient a sense of security and shows respect and courtesy).

    Yes, I think I know how you feel and I see your point of view...however...

    Yes, that's true Mr. Patient. However, let me ask you this one question. If you feel you can't afford the investment today to take care of this one critical tooth and get your other teeth and gums in good condition so this doesn't happen to them....how will you afford it when several other teeth need this same treatment?

5. Confirm that your response or answer was acceptable (again gaining agreement) and then move on.

When the Patient Raises an Objection Due to a Drawback

1. Remind the patient of the benefits he has already accepted or agreed upon.

    Let's take another look at your overall situation... or
    Let's review all the factors involved in your decision... or
    Let's take a look at the investment in detail...

Then go on to:

> When you consider all your needs, Mrs. Jones, isn't (benefits accepted) more important than (the drawback involved)?

> When you consider all these factors, don't you agree that your dental needs (your mouth, your teeth, you) are well worth the investment?

2. If need be, go back and probe for needs again. Find out what the patient's hot button is before trying to proceed and relate treatment back to the patient's hot buttons.

Objections are always known to your patient and not necessarily to you. Sometimes there may be a *hidden objection* that you have not yet identified. If you're not getting full attention...or if you can't seem to smoke out the real objection, ask this question:

> Mrs. Jones, I sense there is something on your mind. (Pause) Can you tell me what it is?

Another situation that involves a different kind of objection is where a patient is coming to you because he wouldn't accept the diagnosis and treatment plan at the last dental office he visited. After you go through the need identification questions, but before you get to the actual exam, you might say:

> You know, Mrs. Jones (smiling and in a friendly tone)...I'm in a bit of a quandary here. You told me when we first started talking that you left your last dentist because he wanted to take x-rays and study models. I can understand your concern because you didn't understand why they would benefit you. The only way I can help you bring your mouth into a healthy condition and keep it that way is to know exactly what I am working with...and that involves doing what you have already told me you don't want to do.

I need to know what is going on in order to know what we need to do. I need x-rays to show me all the bony structures of your mouth to determine if there is any bone loss or periodontal disease, cavities, tumors or cysts, or any abnormalities in the jaw joints. (Continue on depending upon whether or not you will need study models, impressions, ec.)

After we complete this today, we'll schedule you to come back for a consultation appointment in 5-7 days. I'll need some time between now and then to study your situation, including reviewing your study models and x-rays, as well as what my findings are in the clinical exam. Based on that, I will develop a treatment plan which we will discuss in depth at your consultation appointment. When you come back I'll answer anything you want to know about your mouth. I'll tell you exactly what the situation is, what I recommend you do... what I'd do if it was my mouth. If you don't like what I tell you, I'll give you the x-rays and models to take wherever you want to take them. But, Mrs. Jones...your dental health is too important to guess at...and that's why we need to do these things today. How does that sound?

Objections in the Close

When you have fully completed the Principled Selling process and the patient has been involved throughout (and you have gained agreement along the way), you should get a positive response to the treatment plan presentation and acceptance to go ahead. If something is of concern to the patient, by now the patient should feel comfortable enough to tell you. The mutual trust level should be up.

If, however, you are receiving objections in the close, it is usually a sign that:

1. You haven't gathered enough information from the patient along the way to find out what is really important to the patient.

2. You haven't identified needs clearly enough and related the treatment necessary back to the needs, including the patient's wants.

3. You don't have the trust level built up sufficient for the patient to feel comfortable with your recommendations or going ahead with treatment.

4. You have misjudged the patient and have responded in such a way that offended his or her personality style.

5. You have a technical problem or a condition, in which case you have little or no control.

Although having "pat" answers to objections runs the risk of answering a pat answer to a wrong question, there are certain common objections you can think about in advance so you will be prepared with a good response before they arise.

Here are some examples: The patient statement is underlined and a suggested response follows.

I can't afford the whole treatment plan right now.
Mrs. Jones, what would you like to leave out? (usually people don't want to leave anything out!)

My friend had this done by another dentist and it was cheaper
Mr. Smith, we know the value of our dental service and our fees are established accordingly. We also know that the bitterness of low quality lasts much longer than the sweetness of low price.

I need to discuss it with......
Great. Do you feel comfortable conveying your needs and the diagnosis we've discussed so far, or would you like to schedule another appointment and bring (name) with you so I can go over it with him?

What objection do you think he might have to your treatment?

(This gives you an edge in being able to confront and handle any possible objection from this person, or arm the person with information to handle the objection if it comes up.)

That's more than my insurance will cover.
I know you have insurance and I know you may be concerned about whether or not your insurance covers what my recommendation will be. Let me explain to you, however, that I am going to recommend to you optimal treatment and I will base it on what I would do in my mouth. I will not compromise your health by making my diagnosis based on what your insurance company says they will cover.

"We just don't have the money" or "It costs too much."
Note: This could be a condition...but find out. There are several ways to handle it if it is an objection:
If money is an issue, then it would be in your best interests to figure out a way to afford the treatment, Mrs. Smith. You see, left untreated, as we discussed, this could possibly result in _____ which will cost you in the range of ($ to $) to take care of the tooth (teeth) if that happens.

How much too much? (Then listen and when you see what the difference is...say the patient says $100 too much...say) Isn't the extra $100 today worth it so you can keep this tooth?

Is the initial investment your most important concern, or for a few more dollars wouldn't you rather have (then list all the benefits she agreed to and wanted).

Mr. Patient, let me ask you a very important question, and think about it before you respond. Can you really put a dollar value on your health?

Mr. Patient you know as well as I do there is a price to be paid for quality...either you pay for it today...or you'll pay for it tomorrow in reduced results. Which do you prefer?

We can't produce the kind of quality we provide our patients for any less.

The investment you will make is ($ amount) but the benefit and value you will get is the ability to (then list what the patients wants and desires are).

Which is more important to you...long term value and cost effectiveness...or the initial investment and short term value?

I agree with you Mrs. Patient, there is an investment to be made for quality. But when you add the benefits, and eliminate the pain and disappointment of low quality, or no treatment at all, isn't going ahead with this treatment plan really in your favor?

I agree, there is an investment associated with this treatment. But when you consider the ($ amount) isn't it a more than fair trade in order put your natural teeth in healthy condition so you can keep them for a lifetime?

I just don't think so
As a knowledgeable patient your input is invaluable to us. What is it about the treatment plan that doesn't interest you?

I'll think it over
That's fine, Mrs. Patient. Obviously you wouldn't take the time to think it over unless you were seriously interested, would you? Just to clarify my thinking, what is it that you want to think over...is it the:

    ...diagnosis and treatment plan?
    ...the benefits you will receive?
    ...the time involved in having the treatment completed?
    ...the investment (always ask about the fee last)

Or...
If you were going to get started, when would you want to begin ?

Or...
Can you see where this will (list out the benefits she said she wanted)? And are you sincerely interested in (the benefit)? Then I guess I'm not clear, if you understand the benefits...and you understand the consequences if your situation is left untreated...what is it you'd like to think over?

<u>Patient is simply hesitant...and doesn't commit one way or the other</u>
A decision is only as good as the facts...isn't that right? Why don't we list all the pros and cons....(go into the Ben Franklin close).

These are some of the objections you might encounter, and when you do, be glad. By far the toughest patient of all is the agreeable one who offers no objection. This person smiles, nods and gives you all the yeses throughout the entire process and when you ask the closing question says no. There are many ways to respond if this happens. One would be to calmly lean forward and say,

Mrs. Patient, you've agreed all the way through that you have a need (then list the points of agreement on the need), that you feel the benefits (and list the benefits) would solve your problem (take care of your needs). Do you mind my asking why you have decided not to accept the treatment plan that is in your own best interest?

Then don't say another word. Give the patient time to think and respond. Don't you break the silence. The patient will probably do one of two things. She will say, "It's because..." and then give you an objection you can respond to and move on to gain acceptance, or she may say, "What makes you think I'm not going to go ahead with the treatment?" In which case you can proceed with getting her scheduled.

Once you have handled the objections in the close, you might ask one last question in getting to the acceptance of the treatment plan. "Mrs. Patient, is there anything else that would prevent you from beginning your treatment at this time?" When she answers no, then it's time to get her scheduled.

The objections you might encounter are many, but the process for handling them is the same. Before we move from objections, lets make sure we understand two things about patients. *All patients want to be understood and many patients at the time of making a decision are afraid they might make the wrong decision or make a mistake.* Listen to your patients. Make every effort to identify the need, present the solution, and gain agreement all the way through. Be clear about handling objections.

> If a patient truly is a prospect (all four conditions
> present in order to be a qualified prospect),
> there are only two reasons people don't want
> to go ahead with treatment. They don't
> believe it will solve their problem...or
> they don't believe they have a problem.

If you've done the best you know how to do and they still don't buy, don't beat yourself up. Do what you know to do and then move on. Then critique yourself and see where you need improvement and work on doing better the next time. Know, however, that no matter how great you are in the selling process...no matter how good you become in identifying needs, doing the exam and presenting the treatment plan, you probably won't ever get to the place that you sell every single patient, every single time.

Finally, know that your own perceived values, your deepest beliefs, and those of your team...will be transferred to your patient. If you or your team members believe the treatment really is too expensive, if you or they don't believe the treatment really needs to be done, that will be communicated to your patient...verbally or nonverbally. Many patients you think "can't afford it" are eating out, taking vacations, buying new clothes, buying a new car or home entertainment center, or something else. When you understand and believe the value you have to offer, then your patients will too....and not until then. When each of you crosses that line where the value is unquestioned you will see much of the objections you are now encountering dissipate like water evaporating from a sidewalk on a hot day.

Chapter 34

VERBAL SKILLS

A great part of sales ability has to do with verbal skills. What you say is important, but how you say it is just as, if not more, important. If the verbal skills among the team members are weak, it most often follows that treatment plan acceptance is also weak. But communication and verbal skills can be learned right along with the selling skills and the acceptance rate will increase dramatically.

Verbal skills will help you create the mental images and emotional feelings in the patient. This is very significant considering people do not change from their current position unless they feel emotionally moved or disturbed enough to do so. Let's remember this: People do things for one of two reasons...to avoid fear or to fulfill a desire. And people will most often do things first to avoid fear...and move to the other side only when the desire becomes so strong that it overpowers any fear.

Emotions can trigger or destroy
treatment plan acceptance.

Every word you say creates an image in the patient's mind. If you create fear of working with you and your staff, the patient will fight you. Remember that one of the biggest blocks to selling (treatment acceptance) is lack of trust. What you want to do is create an emotional climate that will allow the patient to feel comfortable in accepting your recommendation.

Patients don't remember what you say unless you can create pictures in their minds. Words and their structure within the sentence, and the emphasis we place on them, have great impact. But *word* pictures have even greater impact.

For example, a new patient has obvious infection. During the early phase of the clinical exam, the instant your probing shows symptoms of periodontal disease show the patient. Use your intraoral camera if you have one, or have the patient hold a mirror if you don't, and get the patient involved. Then, rather than saying, "See how far this probe goes?" or "Do you see how the gum bleeds when I put just a bit of pressure on it?" create a word picture and at the same time disturb the patient to build an awareness of his situation. Say something like, "Do you see how the gum bleeds? And can you see the pus oozing from the pocket? It's really amazing that you can have such a serious infection and feel no pain in the diseased area."

Strong? Yes. But is it fair to let your patients off easily, thinking it isn't that big of a problem, and then have them do virtually nothing to correct their problems? It is *your responsibility* to make the situation come alive so your patients will take action. Again, patients don't necessarily remember what you say. They will, however, remember the pictures created in their minds.

Because of this, it is important that we use whatever aids are available to magnify the message in order to make an impact. Creating word pictures by using intraoral cameras, mirrors, picture of patients with similar problems, and any other aids will held people to understand better and become more emotionally involved. Don't shy away from words that evoke emotion such as pus, infection, disease, dead tissue, losing teeth, and requiring dentures or plates. These are words that create visual images and disturbance.

The way we speak with a patient can have a profound effect on whether or not they accept the treatment plan. And it is how you say it that will make the difference. The words we use, our tone of voice, our expressions and our body language all form an impression for our patients. By being aware of the impact we are having, we can make some adjustments and reap rewards for both the patients and ourselves.

Depending upon what mental picture or emotion you are trying to create, you'll want to use different words. For example, if you are in the need identification stage of the selling process and want to *disturb* the patient to move to action, consider using the following:

Say: If we allow this *disease* to *continue to progress*....you *will lose your teeth.*

Not: To keep your teeth we'll need to...

Say: The pain you are feeling with this one tooth you may soon feel with other teeth if we don't take some corrective measures now.

Not: To make you more comfortable we'll need to do...

Say: To give you a brighter smile and whiter teeth, which you've said you want...

Not: We'll do cosmetic dentistry to take care of this for you.

Say: See this pus? It is a sign that periodontal disease is present.

Not: Your gums aren't healthy.

Say: If we don't take care of these teeth immediately we will have to pull them (or extract them) from your mouth and...

Not: If we don't do something we'll need to gently remove the teeth and...

When we are *not* in the need identification stage and are *not* trying to disturb the patient, but rather we want to put the patient at ease, here are some other suggestions for the words we use:

Say: My *professional fee* for these services is...

Not: The *cost (or charges)* for these services is...

Say: If you'll *authorize (or approve)* this agreement...
Not: If you'll *sign this contract...*

Say: This is an *investment* in your health....
Not: This is the *price you must pay* for your health...

Say: What could we improve to make your visit even better?
Not: Was everything all right?

Other words and phrases to stay away from include:

I'm sorry...

Don't apologize unless you truly are meaning to apologize. For example. Let's say you use an answering machine for hours the office is closed. The recording should not begin with "I'm sorry, but our office is closed until...." You don't need to apologize for not working 24 hours a day. Sorry also sets up an unconscious mind set in the patient that perhaps you are not there when you really should be...and consequently they begin to believe that perhaps you don't provide the service they want.

I'll try...

This tells us nothing except that probably you'll use it as an excuse not to get it (whatever it is) done, or that you'll do it if you think of it. Say"*I will* " and then tell what you will do.

I'll try to help you...

Again, this sounds like you might make a half-hearted attempt to help. Say *"I'll be glad to help you."*

I can't...

Instead of telling a patient (or an employee, or doctor) what you can't do, focus on what you can do. Perhaps say, *"I haven't yet, but I can..."* or *"We don't have that option but what I can do for you is..."* Don't concentrate on what you can't do, it places limits and appears that you are not service oriented or don't really want to help.

I failed...
> Instead of looking at anything as a failure, instead consider using the words *I learned.*

No problem...
> Many people say this when someone asks if they can do something or help with something. Instead say *"I'll be happy to do that, "* or *"That's absolutely great."* *"No problem"* actually plants a seed in the mind of the person receiving the message that maybe it really is a problem, or you don't really want to do it, or it really isn't okay.

A number of words have also been identified that act as persuasion words with the general population. These words include:

free	safe	guarantee
health	save	discover
money	easy	proven
new	results	love

Use them in combination to increase the power of the image.

> Follow our *proven* methods and we'll *guarantee* you will have better *results.* You'll *discover* why our patients *love* to visit our office. We make dentistry *safe* and *easy.*

There are also many phrases patients love to hear, including:

> You're entitled to...
> You can rely on us to...
> You can take advantage of...
> You'll be glad to know...
> You can be assured...
> You can depend upon us to...
> Your time is valuable and we respect it.

When we use these phrases with patients they will know we are thinking of them, and they will like it.

Consider, too, how the words you use sound. A good example is "recall." Recall sounds like the person is defective! Isn't that what they do to cars or pieces of equipment with a problem? And what about "cleaning?" It sounds like the person is dirty...and they may conclude that if they brush every day there is no need for a "cleaning."

Fall in love with words. Learn to create word pictures. Word pictures stay with your patients. We must reach the emotional part of our patients before our ideas and treatment plans can be understood and accepted by their rational or thinking self.

The emotional part of a person is sensitive to movement, eye communication, music, types of words used, body language and gestures. Trust, credibility and likability are established here. The emotional connection made here at the unconscious level is then passed to the rational or thinking brain of the patient. Word pictures help us communicate and activate both sides of the brain and cause our patients to not only hear, but also to feel, what we are saying.

Emotional word pictures do five things.

(1)   They focus and direct attention.
(2)   They make the communication come alive.
(3)   They lock what you say, your words, into the patient's memory.
(4)   They are a precursor or pathway to building trust and relationships.
(5)   They will cause a person to act because the communication is deeply felt.

The steps necessary to create a word picture are:

(1)   Know what your purpose is (to clarify, to inform or instruct, to correct, to praise, etc.).
(2)   Find out what the person's interests are (get to know the patient so you can build word pictures that will create emotion and disturbance).

(3)   Draw from life around you...nature, things, stories, history, etc....to develop your word picture.
(4)   Practice the word picture.
(5)   Be persistent.

Some examples that might come up from identifying patients interests are: motorcycles, fishing, hunting, skiing, sewing, parenting, family, animals, racing, golfing, tennis, traveling, art, etc.

Let's look at an example here of how you might use a patient's interest to help you create a word picture and get your point across.

The patient is a pilot. You have discussed the need for a comprehensive exam but he is hesitating a bit, so you say, "Mr. Pilot, not doing a comprehensive exam is like taking off in your plane without filing a flight plan." Or perhaps rather than the exam, your pilot is hesitating about the treatment you recommended. Say something like, "Mr. Pilot, not having this treatment completed is like ignoring your mechanic's advice that your carburetor is faulty and then going into flight knowing the probability is that it will fail you.

Another patient may be a skier who is hesitating about needed treatment. You could say, "Mr. Skier, not having this treatment completed is like not replacing faulty bindings and going ahead and skiing anyway.

Stories, analogies and metaphors are great when they clearly make a point. They can lend credibility to your character, add strength to your presentation and can illustrate your point much more vividly in many cases.

In addition to being concerned about the words and expressions you use, pay attention to your enunciation. How clearly do you speak? Can a patient hear you well, or is it difficult even with the best of hearing to understand what you are saying because you are mumbling, speaking too quickly, or too softly. Speak so you can be heard distinctly, and be sure you use words that most people would understand. Your patients probably won't accept a treatment plan they cannot understand reasonably well.

Power Phrases

Power phrases were mentioned in the discussion about presenting the solution. How you say something can give a totally different meaning, and a startling difference in impact.

Power phrases help you to say better and more effectively whatever it is you want to say. They are excellent tools in the selling process and help us in five areas:

1. They grab the attention of the patient.
2. They keep attention from wandering.
3. They maintain interest.
4. They can be used to answer some objections.
5. They can add punch to the close.

Power phrases are effective ways of expressing a point in a neat, concise, dynamic manner. In a few words they say much more than a drawn out explanation. Every word in the power phrase means something and adds to the impact of the message.

A power phrase must be planned out in advance and delivered in a polished form, not created in front of your patient. The secret of a power phrase, in fact, lies in preparation, planning and practice. They should be phrases you know as well as your own name.

Ben Feldman is widely regarded as the greatest life insurance salesman who ever lived. He was short, stocky, a high school dropout, shy, and had an unmistakable lisp. One fond memory I have of him was at an insurance sales rally I attended (in a large auditorium where several insurance agents from many companies gathered), and Ben spoke standing behind a screen because he was too shy to speak directly to the people attending!

Although he was a man who never finished high school, and wasn't the outgoing individual one might think necessary to be the success he was (he sold $1.6 billion of life insurance in his career), he did his homework throughout his career...literally up until the day he died at age 81 in 1993.

Ben Feldman is the father of power phrases, and he spent hours and hours perfecting his "Feldmanisms" which he so lovingly shared with agents in the life insurance industry through his books, audio tapes and videotapes. It was the power phrases that made Ben stand out. Such as, "The day you walk out, the government walks in, and they want money." or "No one has a lease on life." Others include, "When it comes to settling an estate, women and children don't come first...the creditors do." Or "Here are two checks. This one, the big one, is made out to Uncle Sam. The little one is made out to New York Life. You pay the little one, we'll pay the big one." Or, "The years have a way of making a person old. We have a way of making them secure." Or, "You know that a person runs and runs and they build and build. After a while, they have accumulated a lot of bricks and stones and steel. Then one day they die. Uncle Sam takes it apart overnight. They have a name for it...they call it taxes."

Ben taught me a great deal in the life insurance business, but the principles are just as powerful in dentistry. The difference between the right word and almost the right word is like making the sale and almost making the sale. One gets great results and benefits, the other is close but nothing happens.

Norm gets asked by patients periodically if he will carry an account in house, allowing a patient to string out payments over several months. He has come up with a great power phrase that gets the point across in very few words, "I would rather be your dentist, not your banker." He then lets the patient know that Judy will be happy to discuss the financial options available.

Here are a few power phrases to get you started. Take the time, individually or with your team, to come up with your own.

Quality dentistry isn't expensive...neglect is.

The sweetness of low price never equals the bitterness of low quality.

You'll pay the price either way...there's a price for doing something and an even bigger price for doing nothing.

Mr. Patient, is price your greatest concern...or are you more interested in quality?

Wouldn't you say that your dentistry is worth what it can do for you, not what you have to pay for it?

It is easier to explain our professional fee one time that to apologize for low quality forever.

Take some time to work with power phrases. Your involvement with the patient will really come alive, you'll be much more effective in your selling process, and it will be much more fun. Think about what you say to patients now. Many things you already say could be turned into power phrases with a little work.

Once you have identified some power phrases, write them down, memorize them and don't change them. To change them decreases their impact. At first it may seem like a big feat to accomplish, but stay with it and you'll reap the benefits of your work.

Early in my insurance career I wanted so much to be like Ben, to be the master of power phrases. So, I studied and studied. I borrowed power phrases from others until I could come up with my own. And I simply kept at it.

A few years later, when I was in sales management, one of my agents said, "Cheryl, how did you ever develop all those power phrases and make them sound so easy?" It was then that I realized my hours of study and working through them really paid off. And today? I still use power phrases in every aspect of my speaking, training and consulting career. I'm still putting them together...and I'm sure I will as long as I'm alive.

You can do it too. Learn and perfect your verbal skills by planning and rehearsing until everyone on the team is able to respond to any patient in a positive, nurturing manner. Use power phrases at strategic points throughout your involvement with the patient. When you use a power phrase and give it the right emphasis vocally and tonally, you wake-up the patient and capture attention.

As we said much earlier, selling is about service. That's what you are doing in dentistry...you are serving. You are not just providing dental services, you are building relationships.

A recent 20-year retrospective study of Harvard business school graduates revealed that the most glaring omission in the curriculum was interpersonal skills training. This suggests that the theories of leadership in the past did not anticipate such a great need for building relationships and interpersonal relating in the workplace. This is perhaps much like dental schools not anticipating the dentist's incredible need for practice management and development skills, and leadership skills, and dental teams not understanding the need for relationship building and providing service beyond the actual dentistry for the patient.

Take some time with your team. Discuss how you handle each step of the Principled Selling process. Discuss what kind of behavior gives the impression you want to make, then go the extra mile to make it happen. You'll be surprised, and incredibly pleased, with the results.

Chapter 35

PATIENT RELATIONS

Although you are a doctor of the masticatory system, when you received your diploma you accepted a responsibility that includes much more than that: You are a doctor, a healer. By virtue of your chosen profession you are a doctor of the entire being of that person when they are present to you. Thus, *patient relations* and *customer service*. They go hand in hand with what you want to accomplish clinically, and certainly financially, in your practice.

> One of the essential qualities of the clinician is
> interest in humanity, for the secret of the care of the patient
> is in caring for the patient.
> *Francis Peabody, noted physician and Harvard professor*

Sometimes in the rush of everyday routine and the not so routine, in the face of staff issues and financial concerns, we may forget that patients are people with incredible histories. Some are happy, some are sad. Some have had relatively easy lives while others have suffered substantially. They come to you with many fears: the fear of pain, of losing their teeth, of losing their youthful appearance, of aging, of illness, of suffering, of death...perhaps even angry believing that nature or life has played a cruel trick. They are all human beings who have needs and feelings, and all of them need us to recognize their humanity, dignity, and personal worth. In the rush we may sometimes treat a patient as a specimen, a case number, a crown or a bridge, but not as a person. These people, indeed every person in our practice, need and want our full attention. They want to be cared for, *even when they don't act that way!*

Customer service is a subject much discussed today, and as a result companies abound with mottoes built around "people are our number one interest." Unfortunately, just having a slogan or motto doesn't make it so in reality. Customer service or customer relations, as it is called in other industries, translates into patient relations in dentistry. Satisfied patients are important to the success of your practice, and to the level of enjoyment you experience in your practice. An unsatisfied patient is one of the most expensive, most stressful problems to have!

Patient relations, some would argue, begins at the front desk. I disagree. Patient relations and customer service begin on the *inside*, in your head and in your heart, the same place service begins.

Patient relations is an inside job.

It has to do with your vision and mission, with your values and philosophy of practice, and how they are lived out. Quality patient relations requires and is impossible without service, and true service is not simply an act or series of tasks and behaviors, but an attitude. It is love in action. Quality patient relations begins with you. What employees see modeled is what they will follow...no better, no worse. The kind of relationship you and your team have with your patients will be determined to a large extent by how you treat your employees. Most often, your employees will treat a patient with the same care and consideration that he or she is given by you.

The public has become more and more aware of what they believe to be their rights as consumers, and as a result we are seeing an increase in malpractice suits by dissatisfied patients. The interesting factor here is that many suits are filed not because of poor quality of dental treatment, but because the patients felt they received a poor quality of treatment somewhere else along the line in dealing with the dental office. Dentistry today, because of this heightened awareness of the public, requires much more than the understanding and clinical expertise of dentistry. The people part, the psychology of dentistry and of people in general, is just as important. This means we must deal with the whole person, not just the mouth. When we do, the results are greater and patient compliance is enhanced.

A recent survey reported a rather startling fact. Nearly 50 percent of the patients surveyed expressed dissatisfaction with their current experiences in dental offices. I would be very surprised if any practicing dentist did not agree that patient satisfaction is of the utmost importance in building his or her practice. Yet, if this is a universal belief, why are there so many patients dissatisfied with their dental visits? Another survey shows that 68% of patients who leave do so because of indifference. These, as well as numerous other statistics, magnify the importance of creating strong patient relations in your dental practice if you want to have positive, long-term results. Perhaps the most important reason to build the strong relationships, however, is for the satisfaction you and your team will receive personally from truly communicating, caring, and connecting with your patients.

Unfortunately, many dentists and team members believe that completing dental treatment successfully will equal patient satisfaction. Or perhaps they believe if they get along well with the patient that alone will equal patient satisfaction. Neither is true. The problem lies in what the doctor and team *believe* is service, and what the patients *expect* in the way of service. Most people can't evaluate the exam, diagnosis, or treatment. They haven't been to dental school and they simply can't make a judgment of the quality of dentistry. They can, however, make a judgment about the quality in other areas of the practice.

Good is not good enough if the patient expects more.

Adequate, just getting by, or mediocre isn't good enough anymore...at least not if you want to maintain your current patients and your current market share. And it isn't good enough to look around and see where other dental offices are, check yourself, and say, "we're still ahead so we can just breeze along." Whenever we measure our effectiveness by another, we will be sure to lose out in the long run. While we are doing the checking we are looking over our shoulder, and while we are in that mode we are also decreasing our momentum. Forget what the competition is doing and concentrate on your practice. Give it all you've got and you'll never have to worry about the competition.

If you don't care sincerely and continually about not just meeting their wants and needs, but exceeding them, your patients won't see you as being any better than the dental practice down the road. And they certainly won't fall in love with your practice.

> Patient relations is whatever
> your patients tell you it is.

Perception is the key word here. How a patient perceives you is all there really is. Perception by your patient is his reality, and his feelings and actions will be based on that reality. You may think you've provided excellent service to your patient, but if he doesn't feel that way it doesn't much matter what you think.

Expectations

Connecting with our patients and providing them the quality service they have come to demand in today's world begins by seeing all our involvements with a patient...from every telephone call, to every question, to every time they are in the chair....not just as a random set of experiences, but as a path to building a relationship.

$$\text{Customer Service} = \frac{\text{Performance}}{\text{Expectations}}$$

In other words, performance divided by expectations will give you the level of satisfaction a patient experiences. If a patient expects 100 percent and you deliver 50% percent, they will feel they received only half the value. If, on the other hand, your patient expected 100 percent and you returned 150%, the patient's perception will be much higher: he will feel he received half again as much as he bargained for.

Great customer service or patient relations is not a way
of doing certain things, but a certain way of doing all things.

What is the expectation level of *your* patients? Find out; *ask*
them. Determine what it is. Only when you have determined what
it is can you go about meeting and exceeding those expectations.
Operating in a fog, not really knowing what the expectations are,
is indifference. Indifference may result in angry, unhappy patients
who at some point may choose to take their business elsewhere.
Patients must get the message that you are more critical of how
they are treated (both clinically and otherwise) than they will ever
be. When you get that message across by your actions, you will
have fulfilled, satisfied, happy patients.

So what is it that patients today want? Some of the many factors include:

- to be treated as a person with needs, concerns, fears, wants,
  desires
- a dentist who listens, cares, and has a great chairside
  manner
- easily understood explanations by doctor and staff
- a dentist who cares about the patient's comfort
- a dental staff who also cares about them as a person
  (not just a "case")
- ability to ask questions, have them taken seriously and
  answered
- financial options
- convenient appointments
- minimal waiting time for appointments
- notification when check-ups are due
- dentist's availability for emergencies
- comfortable practice atmosphere
- friendly and courteous staff
- state-of-the-art equipment
- safety - infection control, clean, etc.
- clear (perhaps written) post operative instructions
- a dentist and staff who remain current on technology
  and methods

- knowing the financial obligation in advance of treatment
- perceived value equal to or greater than the fee charged
- convenient for them to access
- adequate parking
- children's area in waiting room (if appropriate to type of practice)
- up-to-date, well selected reading material

These are but *some* of the many, many needs and expectations of patients in general. The important thing for you to do is identify "in specific" what *your* particular patients want and expect, then set about meeting those wants and needs. Involve the patient as a partner in his or her dentistry and do everything you can to help them like the experience of doing business with you. Without asking, however, what *you think* constitutes *liking the experience of doing business with you* may be much different than what *your patients expect.*

It is an established, nurtured relationship that will keep your patients coming back. Money isn't even the critical issue. People want many things from a service provider: they want honesty, respect, responsiveness, and competence. They want to feel you are looking out for their best interests. They want to feel involved in the process, not just having someone do something *to* them.

People will pay for quality, but not just quality in the technical, clinical aspects of dentistry. That quality must be perceived in every other area of the practice as well.

There are many benefits beyond satisfied patients when customer service or patient relations is rated high. Practices that provide quality patient service keep their patients longer, have lower marketing costs, experience a higher case acceptance rate, produce a higher amount of dentistry per patient, and have higher net profits. A side benefit is that when the patients are happier, the employees are happier. They tend to stay with their jobs longer and are more satisfied with their jobs.

Quality control is knowing what your patients want and then exceeding those wants. When you use the term "quality" in your practice, whether it be communicating it to your patients or communicating within the team, what does it really mean? Be able to explain it in explicit detail.

> Quality is what your
> patients tell you it is.

Quality to one person on your team may be entirely different from what the next believes to be quality. There must be clear agreement on quality if you are all going to be in the same boat, rowing in the same direction, complementing each others efforts instead of working against each other. Once you are clear on what it means to your patients and to all your team members, then you can provide that quality for your patients. And, when you have a belief system built around it, you will be more likely to communicate it to the patients with such impact that it will be remembered.

Moments of Truth

It is critically important that the entire team be aware of the moment of truth concept. Every contact with the patient, either in writing, over the phone, or in person, is a moment of truth.

> Patient satisfaction is built
> one moment of truth at a time.

The process never ends. Aristotle once said, "Excellence is an art won by training and habituation. We are what we repeatedly do. Excellence, then, is not an act, but a habit."

How you handle moments of truth will set you apart from other practices. Here are several moments of truth that affect your patient relations and satisfaction:

Availability and Responsiveness
- How accessible are you by phone? Does a patient get an answering service or machine? How many rings before the phone is answered?
- When a person calls, are they treated as an interruption or as a welcomed caller?
- How quickly do you return phone calls?
- How quickly does/can a patient receive emergency treatment?
- How long is a patient kept waiting for their appointment?

- How quickly and accurately are questions regarding financial matters handled?
- How is a person asked to be put on hold...and how long are they kept there?
- Are your patients greeted immediately when they enter your office, or is the receptionist involved in a phone conversation (business or personal) and acknowledges the arriving patient only after she is off the phone?

Courtesy, Respect and Care
- Is each patient thanked as he or she leaves the practice?
- Is every team member friendly with the patients?
- Are you available for the patient?
- How do you care for the patient's belongings? (purse, coat, etc.)
- Do you address patients by the name or title they prefer?
- Are you aware of the patient's time and consider it valuable?
- Do you extend special services as a courtesy, including comfort and convenience, such as a telephone or refreshment beverages?
- Do you call following a difficult procedure to check on the patient's progress and comfort?

Credibility
- Do you deliver what you say you will?
- Are you and your team trustworthy, believable and honest?
- Does the patient perceive you to have his/her best interests at heart?
- Do you refrain from criticizing another dentist or his/her work?
- Do you have modern, up-to-date equipment?

Reliability
- Does the job get done right the first time?
- Do you keep your promises...do what you say you will do when you say you will do it?
- Do you handle complaints or problems immediately?

Security
- Does your patient feel secure? What do you do to establish this feeling?
- Is your patient free from doubt? Do you explain the treatment so he/she can understand it and clarify the financial aspects before going ahead?
- Does your patient feel safe physically (free from danger of x-rays, hazardous chemicals, infectious diseases, etc.)? (How do you know the patient is comfortable and feeling safe?)
- Do you and your team refrain from talking about your patients outside the office (confidentiality issue)?

Communication
- Do you listen to your patients...and do they feel listened to?
- Do you check to make sure you understand what you think the patient is saying?
- Do you show that you are interested and concerned about your patients?
- Do you give patients your undivided attention while you are with each of them?
- Do you refrain from judging the patients questions and giving "flip" answers, or in any way diminish respect for the question?
- Do you refrain from speaking "across" the patient to your team members, as though the patient wasn't there?
- Do you communicate in a language the patient can understand?
- Do you let your patient know ahead of time what you are going to do, rather than have it be a surprise?
- Do you deal positively with the control issue? Many patients feel out of control in the dental chair and need the option of being able to communicate that they want you to stop for a moment...essentially allowing them the feeling of control.

Appearance
- Are hairstyles reasonable and well groomed?

- Are you and your team members well groomed and professional in appearance?
- Do each of the team members refrain from too much make-up, cologne or after-shave, gaudy nail polishes, etc.

Each of these questions provides the opportunity to measure your customer service/patient relations levels in your practice. Since *quality doesn't improve unless you measure it*, it is good to regularly go through the questions together to determine how well you are doing.

The consistency of these moments of truth is important. We've heard many times that we never get a second chance to make a first impression...but we must take that even further. We never get a chance to *erase* an impression at any stage of the relationship. People don't forget. We can overcome, but we seldom forget. Therefore, the first impression we make, as well as the last and every one in between, is vitally important. Every patient, every day, must leave your practice feeling satisfied with your service and liking the experience of doing business with you and your team.

Full Circle to Marketing

Once again, we come back to marketing. Everything we do is marketing. When people like the experience of coming to you, when you have integrated them into your practice, they will then refer their family and friends. Remember, the patient chose to come to you...so you begin the relationship on a somewhat positive note. Don't blow the opportunity when they arrive!

In one of my recent travels involving two "legs" on a major airline, I had the experience of observing two totally different teams of flight attendants in action. The first leg of the trip was fun, and made so by the interaction of the attendants. They worked as a team. They seemed to have a mission of truly taking care of and making the flight experience of the passengers an excellent one. They were friendly to each other. I could feel the concern, the courtesy, and the respect they had for each other. It translated into behavior and actions with the passengers that was superb. They served us promptly, were very attentive to the concerns of individual passengers, and asked if there was anything they could do for us.

Everything was done in a manner that said, "I really care. Is there anything I can do to make you more comfortable...to make your flight more enjoyable?" Not only did I enjoy the flight, but I actually enjoyed watching the flight attendants at work!

The next leg was a totally different picture. The flight attendants had little to say to each other, and little to say to the passengers as well. There were no smiles, no laughter, no fun in flight! When the flight attendant came by with the beverage service I asked for a cup of water. By her response, I felt I had really imposed upon her. When we debarked the plane, there were no attendants at the door greeting the passengers as they left. Had this been my only experience of flying I would certainly think twice about flying this airline again.

This example also speaks strongly and boldly about the mission being *communicated to* and *accepted by* the employees, each and every one of them, and to their belief in that mission and desire (or unwillingness) to live it out in their actions for their customers.

> I slept, and I dreamt that life was all joy.
> I woke, and saw that life was but service.
> I served, and discovered that service was joy.
> *Rabindranath Tagore*

Moments of truth must be lived one patient at a time, one moment at a time, day in and day out, every single day. Every moment of choice becomes a moment of truth. We may want to pass off our actions because of something someone said or did, or the circumstance that "made you do it," or the upsetting news or phone call you just received, or the fact that you are angry or upset because the last two patients canceled, but the bottom line is that we are the only person responsible for our actions, and the quality thereof. We discussed employees in part two. Review this section regularly. Understand that only an encouraged, empowered team can serve your patients well and in the manner that allows excellence of service. This alone will make a big difference between you and the dental practice down the street.

Let's look at an example of a moment of truth outside normal practice hours.

It's late Friday afternoon, you are getting ready for a ski trip the next day and you're in the middle of putting the ski rack on your vehicle. Your spouse answers the phone and tells you it is a patient calling because his temporary crown just came off. Because you're right in the middle of placing the ski rack on your vehicle you say, "Tell Mr. Jones I'm right in the middle of putting my ski rack on the car. Get his number and tell him I'll call him as soon as I'm through.

No big deal, you say? Think again. Not only will the patient feel like he is a "nuisance or interruption" but he may also feel that he isn't as important as your ski rack. To you, it's no big deal. To the patient it is a very big deal.

We must develop the habit of continual improvement. We must develop the habit of listening to our customers, of listening to each other, of being creative and innovative as we strive to meet the needs, wants, desires, and expectations of our patients. Today's patients expect high quality and customized service. That means our practice teams must pay attention to detail. It means we must respond to our patients' needs with courtesy and knowledge. They want quality, and affordability, not either/or, or a compromise between the two. We must continually ask two questions: *(1) How are we doing?* and *(2) What and how can we do better?*

Perception really is all there is! Quality patient relations and customer service is how you perform from your patients' point of view. The road to mediocrity begins with that first compromise...don't do it. To do this we must remember that it begins with the practice team. You must provide them with a service they can encourage, sell and support with pride. When you do, you will be on the road to providing patients with quality and satisfaction. Remember, nothing positive happens for your patients until you or another team member does it. Awareness of these moments of truth is critical...excellence is critical.

The Pulse of Your Practice: Patient Input

So how do you really know what your patients' perceptions are? How do you really know what you are doing? Remember, only 4 out of 100 people who stop doing business with you will ever tell you why.

Input from your patients is important, and many of the best ideas on how you can improve your service will come directly from them. We sometimes get so concerned about the output that we forget about the input! We need to make friends with customer complaints as well, so we can learn from them. There are several ways to get this input.

Unsolicited input from patients is valuable. Unfortunately, many do not offer this kind of input. When you do receive it, however, take a close look at what you are hearing before you throw it away as unfounded. Check it out. Talk with each other as a team. Discuss what could have caused the perception...and how you can do better the next time. Or, if the input is really great...discuss that too. Make sure everyone on the team understands clearly what it was that led to that positive comment. And then commit to doing more of it more often.

Questionnaires. Surveys or questionnaires are one form to gather or generate input about your practice from your patients. One method is to have these forms available for patients to complete when they are in your office. Another is to mail the form to all your patients with the return postage included. Either way, let them know you want their opinion about the treatment they receive in your dental practice so you can continually improve your response to their needs and desires.

In our practice we have a specially designed and hand-crafted oak comment box that my father made for the practice. It speaks of quality with its solid oak construction, hand carving, and brass plate that reads "We value your comments. J. N. Matschek, D.M.D." On either side of the comment box are holders for the patient comment cards with several questions to be completed by the patient.

It is certainly much easier, and less expensive, to keep a patient than to gain a new one. We cannot, must not, take patients for granted or we will have to keep finding new ones to replace the ones we lost, as well as needing new ones to replace the natural attrition that occurs because of moving, death, and simply for those who are dentally healthy and return for maintenance only.

Focus groups are another source of patient perception and information regarding your service. Focus groups typically involve from six to eight people at a time, with no more than ten, all brought together around a central topic or question. The question might be a very specific one, such as *How can we better meet your needs as they relate to your appointments, schedule, and availability?* Or the focus group might meet around a more general question such as *How can we better serve your needs and make your experience in our practice a positively remembered one?*

It is important that you provide a benefit for patients who serve on the focus groups. Perhaps you might want to provide dinner for those involved, whether it be at a local restaurant or bring in pizza or something appropriate and meet in your staff lounge or conference room. Maybe you prefer to offer a special courtesy discount on their next appointment, or maybe you could provide them with a gift certificate for tickets to a movie, dinner, sports event or some other appropriate entertainment.

Regardless of the method you choose to get patient feedbck, two questions should be kept in mind: *(1)What do you like?* and *(2)How can we do better?*

In order for your service to be remembered as outstanding, you and the entire team must be committed to service. Each must recognize the need for, and maintain, a continuous improvement philosophy. You must listen to your patients, as well as suppliers, and act on ideas you receive that are of benefit. It must be clear what the rules of the game are, so to speak (values, beliefs, commitments) so everyone can be successful. Every team member should be held accountable for providing excellent service and there should be some measurement of performance from the patients' point of view. Then, finally we must remember to celebrate our successes. We must make the practice a fun place to be.

Typically we see that excellence of service is most often found where the team members say their doctors have a strong commitment to service and back it up with their behavior and actions. Interestingly, turnover and morale among employees closely correlates with the patients' satisfaction of the service quality provided. It is important to understand that your team members are very conscious of what you, as doctor and leader, do. They listen to what is being preached or espoused, and then watch for action and behavior to support that. In other words, *how* you do what you do is as important as *what* you do. This means that the Personal and Professional Development Sessions mentioned in part two have a strong, double need. Feedback must be given not only on technical quality, but on interpersonal style and skill as well. Obviously this requires that you (or your office manager or supervisor) pay attention to how the employee is doing, and then evaluate and give feedback. This is missing in many dental offices. The receptionist who puts together great financial agreements but leaves the patient feeling cold and uncared for isn't providing quality service. The assistant that takes great x-rays but treats the patient abruptly or hurriedly will also leave the patient feeling uncared for.

Translate clearly and discuss with your team what quality means in your practice. Identify specifically what it looks like in behavior. What is your mission? How does that translate into behavior? What does it look like in action? Regardless of the position of the team member in the practice, it is imperative that each person keep their focus and consciousness high about total patient care. Service quality doesn't just happen at the front desk, or chairside. It either happens throughout the practice, by every employee in every position, including the doctor, or it doesn't happen at all. The experience the patient will remember is the total experience. If any part of that experience doesn't meet the patients expectations, the entire experience will be chalked up to one that he doesn't feel comfortable or good about, or want repeated. Perhaps it wasn't a terrible experience, it was okay or so-so...but again, that's not good enough. When someone tells your patient about the wonderful experience they had down the street you want to be in a position that your patient doesn't say, "Gee, maybe I ought to give it a try" but instead says, "Nothing could equal *my* dental office. You ought to give *them* a try!"

Chapter 36

COMMUNICATION: WHAT MESSAGE ARE YOU SENDING?

Patient relations is one reason communication is important, but there is another aspect involving communication and patient relations that is vitally important. I doubt there is a dentist around who doesn't shiver at the utterance of malpractice, liability, or OSHA. As a result, risk management continues to be high on the list of priorities for consideration and discussion....and it involves communication.

We are facing a public that is growing more aware of its rights (what has come to be called "rights") as consumers of healthcare, as well as a growing number of malpractice suits by dissatisfied patients. Legal counsel indicates communication is where the relationship is established and grown, or breaks down and causes people to think litigation. Today, just as we must be aware of new technology, new materials and methods, we must also become masters of the interpersonal skills so necessary in developing a healthy, positive, patient/doctor relationship. That means that an effective practice today almost assuredly requires an understanding of psychology and communication, as well as dental science.

Communication is the most powerful tool in dentistry today. Allen Thomas, from Thomas and Fees (a California accounting firm specializing in dentists) says, "We know from experience that the formula for a financially successful dentist is 10 percent clinical ability, 20 percent business savvy and 70 percent communication skills." Dr. Maurice Teitlebaum (Dental Economics, February 1992) puts it this way, "For the most part, the reason patients leave a practice is a result of the failing of a dentist in his/her relations with a patient." Patients are sensitive to relationships: their relationship with you; their relationship with your team; and the relationships between the team members, including you. How are you and your team coming across to your patients?

No two practices are exactly alike, and because this is true, the methods, procedures and organizational styles that work in one office won't necessarily be as effective in the next. Personality, objectives, goals, and values all contribute to the uniqueness of each person and practice. There is a need for one common denominator, however, and that is effective communication. A number of principles apply to all communication. These principles, when specifically applied to the dental practice, will help create an atmosphere of trust, and build relationships that will minimize the possibilities of malpractice suits and the litigious mentality.

It is helpful to remind ourselves regularly what communication involves. It is the process of *sending* and *receiving* messages and exchanging verbal and nonverbal thoughts, opinions, information, and self-revelation. Self-revelation? Yes! Only 15 percent of communication is verbal. The other 85 percent is nonverbal. By your communication, both verbal and non-verbal, you reveal to others much of who you are...even what you think you are hiding! And herein lies the key message for communication and how it relates to the litigious mind. Communication is hearing with all the senses and checking perceptions. Although we learn to *speak* and to *hear*, very few people are taught to *communicate* and to *listen*.

Two major problems commonly occur in communication. The first is *assuming everyone is in the same place we are.* The second is *assuming they have the same frame of reference.* Many erroneous ideas and false beliefs are generated because people do not have the understanding about what occurs in dentistry that you and your team do. So, the first reaction of many is to believe everything they see or hear. They simply do not have the same frame of reference or come from the same background as you.

Very briefly, let's identify a few of the factors that affect communication...how your message is being sent, as well as how it is being received. These factors form barriers or filters (screens) that your message must go through, and then it must be translated by the receiver through his or her filter system. Here's just a few: self-esteem, attitudes, personality, gender, intellectual acumen, age, expectations, values, language associations, health, prejudices, ego, vocabulary, body language, anxieties and fears, background (experiences), cultural background, voice (tone, rate, etc.), hidden agendas, and the list could go on and on. When you send a message, it is sent based on all this about you. And when it is received, it is received by a person with an intact set of his or her own filters.

For example, if you mention to a patient that a root canal is needed, and that patient has never had a root canal, but has been told by someone else how awful and painful they are (and the patient is white-knuckled just having a prophy completed) you can expect this patient is going to be a bit uptight. On the other hand, if this patient has had an uneventful root canal in the past, or has never had one but has been told by a friend that they're a "piece of cake," it is likely his or her response would be much different.

It is important we understand that what we say is colored, motivated, and influenced by divergent biographies made up of all the factors listed above, and more. Yet these biographies go unacknowledged for the most part.

We are beings controlled by our emotions, feelings and fears. It would be great if communication was translucent so that as we spoke, or hear another speak, our minds were perfectly revealed so the words would register and move through the barriers and filters without any change of meaning in the mind of the other. But this isn't the case.

This implies much for a dental practice. What do you assume your patients know, that they may have no knowledge of? Or what message are you sending that you are unaware of? One dental group's newsletter carried this message for emergency care: *"Our office policy is that we will do our utmost to see patients in discomfort as soon as possible."* Again, what message are you sending by your communication and the communication of your staff? And is it coming across the way you intend for it to be received? Experts on relationships indicate the number one reason for failed relationships is poor communication. This has much meaning for our dental practices.

Most every dentist would agree that the message they want to relate to their patients is *The Four C's*: care, concern, compassion, and competency. But that isn't always the message we are sending, even when we think we are.

Let's look at some key factors in creating the atmosphere for good, healthy communication in the dental office. The most important factor to be clear about initially is that *you, the dentist, set the office tone.* How you relate, respond and communicate sends a message to your team as to what you expect them to be or do. They will follow your lead. It won't work to tell them to be patient-oriented, kind, compassionate, friendly, and positive if you are more concerned about the dollar than the patient, if you lack compassion, or if you are unfriendly or negative.

Have a desire and be willing to listen. All the principles of good communication won't do a thing unless you have a *willingness* to really communicate with your patients...and your staff.

Listen to your patients. Listen when they speak to you face-to-face, when they voice complaints in person or in writing, when they respond to a survey or questionnaire, when they participate in focus groups, when you or any member of your team is educating them to some aspect of dentistry or dental care, when you conduct formal research. Listening is powerful and can give you exactly what you need to make the minor (or major) adjustments in your practice to maintain your patient orientation and continue providing quality that is perceived as such by your patients.

It should be noted that communicating with your team is *just as important* as communicating with your patients. Poor communication or a lack of, in either case, will cause the door you want open to slowly close. Again, because of the verbal and non-verbal communication (body language included), you will be sending messages to patients and team members that you may not even be aware of communicating. The quickest way to turn this around is to reevaluate how you feel about your patients, your team and yourself. When the patient or team member really does become important to you, then the desire will also be there to begin practicing, on a daily basis, the principles for good communication.

Pay attention to the office atmosphere. When you enter your reception area, what does it say about you? If the patient drew his or her total impression about your practice from this area, what would it say about values? What would it tell them about how you feel about your patients? About where your priorities lie? About the kind of dental services they will be receiving? Just what does your physical space communicate? Does it foster a relaxed, non-threatening, comfortable feeling? Is it neat and clean? Does your reception area feel warm and inviting...or sterile? Take a walk through your front door and view it from the patient's perspective. What message is being communicated? Would a patient feel welcomed? And what about how your patients are greeted? Does your receptionist greet the patient immediately with a smile? Or does she have her back turned, filing patient charts, and greet the patient only upon completion of the task? What about the pictures on the wall, are they straight? Do you have any burned out lights? Are the magazines neat, or torn and coverless? And are they current? Is there debris on the floor?

Think about the message your patients are receiving through their five senses. Office cleanliness, music quality and volume, aroma, temperature, magazines, other materials, cleanliness of patient restrooms, work areas (cluttered or clean), appearance of equipment, waiting room, operatories, consultation rooms, you name it...all these physical aspects speak loudly to your patients about how you feel about them and your practice.

What message does your office send to your patient *clientele?* If you have an older, more mature practice, does your environment welcome this type of person...or are you supposedly catering to the elderly clientele, but outfitting your practice for the early adult?

Be sincere...be real. The message you send about compassion, caring and concern will be colored by your sincerity or lack of. People can see through the put-on's. If you really don't care about your patients, they will feel it. The same is true for your team.

Relate to the patient as a person. It is easy to slip into thinking of a patient as the "large reconstruction case" or the #30 crown, rather than Mary Smith or Tom Brown. No one likes to be thought of as a number or a case. If you speak about a patient in front of another patient this way, he has no information to think you would do any differently about him.

Respect the patient's time. This includes not keeping the patient waiting. If it becomes necessary for a patient to spend more than five to ten minutes in the reception area, the patient should be told why and how long it will be. This is common sense and basic respect. If your office schedule gets off track, or you've had an emergency situation arise, have your receptionist call the scheduled patients and have them come in a bit later, or reschedule if necessary. The patient will get a message loud and clear as to whether or not you feel their time is important. This is becoming more and more of a concern in practices today. People expect more than they did in the past, and they expect us to respect their time, just as we expect them to respect ours.

Resolve complaints, misunderstandings about care, the bill, or other matters of concern before the patient becomes resentful. It is true that 95 percent of patients who are unhappy or dissatisfied never say a word...they just leave. Therefore, it makes good sense to listen to the 5 percent who do voice their dissatisfaction. Obviously, not every complaint will be a valid one, but you can be sure that every complaint must be dealt with as though it is. Otherwise you will receive plenty of publicity....but of the variety you would rather not have! I frequently remind dental teams that some of the strongest supporters come from patients who voiced a complaint and who were communicated with immediately, and in a manner that let them know their concerns were important. These people will be happy and stay with you forever, knowing that if there is a problem you will deal with it rather than run away from or ignore it.

Address patients in the manner they wish to be addressed. It is important to refer to a patient by the name they wish to be called. To address an elderly person by their first name before they have given you the okay to do so is in poor taste, and not respectful. Likewise, if a person's name is Kathleen, it is not good to assume she wants to be called Kathy. Find out what the "preferred name" is, and then address your patient this way. The sweetest sound to most people is the sound of their name, so once you find out what they want to be called, use it often.

Stay approachable. This does not mean to have an open door policy that people can enter at any time. What it does mean is that you have an open attitude to having your patients communicate freely with you about their concerns, questions, needs, fears, etc. This approachability will come through quickly if it is there and it helps establish an atmosphere that feels "safe." Most patients, and even family members, want to know that if they do have a question, if they don't understand something, if they just need reassurance, you'll be there. Obviously, this includes returning phone calls. Although this isn't usually on the top of the "like to do" items on a to-do list, returning calls is important. Doing so as promptly as you can sends a message to the patient. First, it says that you care. Secondly, it says they are important and you are concerned about whatever it is that concerns them. Third, it is just plain respectful and good business to do so. Obviously, calls relating to front office matters should be handled by the appropriate personnel, and those calls should be identified before they end up on your desk in the form of a "return phone call" note.

Respect patient confidentiality in all situations, even in social situations. That may seem terribly obvious, but it still occurs repeatedly that a patient's name slips when a doctor or team member is socially involved with peers or friends. Something as simple as going out for lunch with the team members and mentioning a patient's name can create situations where confidentiality is compromised.

It is so easy to end up saying to another person, whether that person is a member of your team, a patient, a patient's spouse or parent, "You misunderstood me" and place blame. And you probably have that thrown back at you at times too. A great communicator, however, knows he or she must take responsibility for what is being communicated, and then assist the other person receiving your message to understand you.

It isn't so much what you *say* as you go about your practice, but what others *hear*. It is *perception, perception* and more *perception*. Legal counsel for our local Dental Association indicates that many dentists think the question in litigation is, "Did I practice good dentistry?" Not true, they say. Much of litigation is involved with appearances and perceptions. The real question one must ask him or herself is, "Did I care?" The legal counsel further indicates, "If the dentist doesn't care and thinks he/she can cover it up, a surprise will be in store. Give that dentist two to three days in front of a jury on a malpractice suit and the message of whether or not the dentist cared will come through loud and clear."

Communication is definitely a most valuable tool in dentistry that can work *for* you. Unfortunately, it can also work against you when you do not pay attention to how you are coming across. In the next chapter we will address ten steps to help you solidly establish a relationship with your patients that will bring you both great rewards.

Chapter 37

COMMUNICATION: ONE TO ONE

Once the principles involved in creating the kind of atmosphere you want are understood, these next ten steps will help you to solidly establish a relationship with your patients that will bring you both great rewards. Your patients will feel great about the experience of having you do their dentistry, and you will feel great because you will have happy, satisfied patients who will return again and again. It will help you establish an atmosphere that is conducive to building trust and therefore positive patient relations, as well as eliminate or reduce the possibility of litigious thinking.

Identify patient needs and wants. It's true that if you show a person what they want, they will move heaven and earth to get it. The only way to identify needs and wants is to ask questions, as we discussed in the previous chapters on sales. This gets the patients involved. Encourage *them* to ask questions and then *really* listen. You want them to talk to you about their wants and their perceived needs. When they ask questions or comment, and you want to know more, keep them going by responding with "That's a very good question..." or "Tell me more..." Remember, people like their own ideas best. Find out how they feel about their dental health, their appearance, their desire to keep their teeth throughout their life, etc. Ask the questions, and when they give you the answers you can relate your diagnosed treatment needs back to what is most important to them. This entire process will help the patient understand that you do care, that you are concerned about what they want, and that you will listen.

Speak their language. Speak with your patients based on their level of understanding. One thing you cannot do in a dental practice is to wait for just the right moment to give the patient information. It's not like waiting until you feel the "time is right" to share something with your husband, wife, or significant other. You must give the news to the patient when he/she is in your office, and it may not be the very best time simply because of the patient's state of mind. However, you can do the next best thing, and that is to *speak to them based on their understanding.* This means not using technical dental terms that mean nothing to the patient. It also means not talking down to them, possibly having them feel you think they are stupid or ignorant, and jeopardizing your relationship with them. Many patients feel uncomfortable, uneasy, and tense while in the dental chair and their ability to really listen is not at a peak. Therefore, speaking their language becomes very important in helping them understand what is going on and what needs to be done.

People normally remember one-third or less of what they heard 24 hours earlier. Logic tells us that even less will be remembered if the patient is frightened, nervous, or in an otherwise agitated state. Therefore, when speaking to a patient of their condition or proposed treatment, be sure to communicate clearly, accurately, and with vivid images as much as possible. Creating vivid word pictures in their minds helps build an association that will stay with them much longer than words, thereby increasing retention. Use pictures as you are explaining to them what has happened to a particular tooth and what needs to be done. Use your intraoral camera or give them a hand held mirror and show them in their own mouth.

Give your undivided attention to the patient you are with at the moment. Ghandi once said, "No matter where you are, be sure you are there." This means to listen, *really listen*, when your patient speaks. Then respond to show you are listening. Be sensitive to your patients' feelings and reflect them back to show your concern.

Your patient, who has just been told she needs a root canal, begins to visibly tense. Hands clench, eyes widen and the faces whitens. She may say, "Do I really have to have that?" and you can see that she is scared. You might respond with, "Carol, have you ever had a root canal?" or if you know that She has and it wasn't by you, "What has been your experience with root canals in the past?" Then it comes out. She's really afraid. The last one was a terrible experience and she hasn't forgotten it. Now it's time for you to respond in a way that let's her know you've listened and you are concerned. "Carol, I can see how much this upset you the last time and I can understand your concern and hesitation based on that experience." Then go on to tell her how you will handle the situation and how you expect it to be different than the last time.

Whatever the situation, give your patient your undivided attention. Invest the time to educate them so they will be in a better position to do their part of the equation.

> **Make the patient the most important
> person in your life at that moment.**

This requires communication which means two-way...not talking *at* the patient, but *with* the patient. It means giving input and receiving input. It means eye contact. It means being sincerely interested in the patients' questions or comments. Without this kind of attention your patients may respect you as the dentist, but they may not like the experience of doing business with you. When this is the result, *they will not be satisfied patients.* Even if they don't leave the practice, they may be the ones who don't make it easy on your or your team, who perhaps routinely show up late or cancel at the last minute, and certainly won't give referrals. When you do give your undivided attention, your patients actually will enjoy coming into your office. So few people today give anyone their undivided attention. Just like thank you's, it is so rare that it will be remembered, and you will be remembered as a great dentist. Your patients' experiences with you will be great as a result.

Dentistry is a people business, and building relationships insures the success of the practice. If the dental team projects a negative attitude creating a negative work environment, the patients will feel it. When the attitude is one of "Welcome, we're glad you're here," when it is not what your patients can do for you but what you can do for them, then you're on your way to building good relationships.

Remembering your patients' concerns will also let your patients know you are really concerned about them and your attention is focused on their well-being. Designate a spot in the chart to make notes to individualize your interaction with each patient. If a patient likes to be called by a nickname, indicate it in the chart and then use it. If the patient has a favorite hobby, be sure to note that and ask the patient what he/she has been doing in that area since the last visit. Perhaps the patient was just leaving for a special vacation when he was last in. Remember to ask about it. Maybe your patient has a specific expectation or concern. Write it down so you'll remember it the next time.

My mother is somewhat claustrophobic and has a difficult time with a rubber dam during treatment. When Norm first treated her and found this out, he made a hole in the rubber dam and immediately lessened her fear. Now, every time she is seen and a rubber dam is used the "hole" is made immediately without question. Mom appreciates this and knowing she doesn't have to ask every time makes her more comfortable.

Be interested. Let your patient know you really care. The principle is so important...people don't care how much you know until they know how much you care.

Watch your body language. It is easy to send conflicting messages to a patient: a message may verbally convey one thing (what you say) and non-verbally communicate something else. Remember, as much at 85 percent of what you communicate is non-verbal. Consider your posture; it reveals a great deal about you. The confident person sits up straight, holds their head up, walks upright, and generally sends out a message that he or she feels good about him or herself. People who lack that confidence often carry themselves in a way that says they don't feel confident.

Eye contact is another non-verbal. Be sure when you speak to your patients that you look directly at them, and not at the floor, the ceiling, the walls, or down into your lap. It has been proven that people feel they can trust people much easier if the person will look directly at them when speaking. Those who don't make eye contact tend to communicate, "There is something I am hiding from you that I don't want to tell you, have you see, etc." It has been said that our eyes are our windows to the soul. Use them wisely in your practice and you'll be building relationships that will last as long as the patient is around and you are in practice.

Another aspect of non-verbal communication is physical contact. In these days of lawsuits and sexual harassment issues, caution must be observed. Nevertheless, many research studies have revealed that physical touch calms people. In your practice you probably already know the ones you can pat on the back or gently squeeze on the arm. But what about the others? A simple but firm handshake is an easy physical contact. It is virtually non-controversial, yet it makes physical contact and creates good feelings.

Finally, what about facial expression? Think about what the patient may see as he is staring into your face while you are doing dentistry. Every time you frown or grimace, the patient may take that for you not liking what you see, that you don't really know how to handle the situation, or any number of other translations. Remember, you are trying to build relationships and put people at ease. Don't make the mistake of thinking that a frown now and then is no big deal. It could well be the one thing a patient picks up on and feels uncomfortable about...maybe uncomfortable enough to seek out another dentist. Perhaps the worse part is that you may never know why. The patient just leaves.

Don't judge. This means to respect the patient and his or her right to refuse your recommendations. Even after you do your very best communicating what the patient needs, or what the patient should do, he may not comply. Try not to criticize. It is important the patient understands the probable results if they do not comply, but they also need to feel they do have the right to refuse treatment without being lectured, harped at, or jumped on.

Don't criticize another dentist's care in front of the patient. There will be times when you see work that is less than the standard of care. The issue here is to keep any comments you make factual and objective. Don't bring personalities into it. Never respond, "Geez, who did this work?" Instead say, "As a result of my examination I find..." and then go on to factually, and as objectively as you can, report your findings. If your patient says, "Well, Dr. Doit did it," and it's something that needs to be redone, you may want to offer to call the treating dentist in that situation and see if he wants to redo it, or have you do it and send him the bill.

We all know there are many contributing factors that affect the quality of the dental work, which may make it appear the work wasn't done to the very best standard. Perhaps the patient was extremely difficult, or is unable to open her mouth sufficiently to do the very best work possible.

Be aware of your tone of voice, and how you emphasize what you say. This is another non-verbal communicator, but it's important enough to discuss separately. We can say almost anything, but with a sarcastic tone what might have been a compliment can turn into a nasty, cutting remark. This is important to remember when speaking to your team, as well as the patient. If a patient senses sarcasm, disagreement or friction with you and your team, or between other team members, this, too, can set up in his mind a question about whether or not this is the place he wants to be. Sarcasm, cutting and biting words, and negativity all cause people to feel uncomfortable. It can translate beyond that, though, to a question of your actual credibility and capability as a dentist. Patients expect professionals to act as professionals. If they don't, they'll wonder just how "professional" the entire organization is.

Ask only yes and no questions when you are working in a patient's mouth. It is extremely embarrassing for some patients to be asked a question when they can't respond. It's interesting to note that people with low self-esteem will often be the ones who feel uncomfortable when they are asked to do something and they can't do it...i.e., they are asked a question by you that can't be answered with a simple yes or no. Even that is difficult to get out when your mouth is otherwise engaged!

Choose your words carefully. Be concerned with what might be misunderstood as well as with what is understood. What does the patient know? What does the patient understand? What might they misunderstand? How might they misinterpret what you want to communicate? How can you avoid this? Remember, what you know very well and have spent many years in education and practice to understand, others do not understand. Ask yourself the question, "Given all I know about this person, how might I expect him or her to receive this message?" Then respond based on your answer.

Further, don't show surprise or bewilderment in front of the patient for some unexpected turn of events during your treatment. Comments like, "Gee, I didn't expect to find this..." or "I wonder why this doesn't fit..." or "I can't imagine how..." or "I can't figure this one out" all may cause the patient to become uncomfortable, nervous, or frightened. This is compounded and made even worse when no clarification is forthcoming and the patient just lays there wondering what in the world is happening.

Be aware that you set the tone in your office. This has been said many times now, but remember that your employees will get their cue from you as to how they are to respond and what they are to do. You may tell them to have a positive attitude, a caring attitude, and a patient-oriented approach, but if you don't exhibit this behavior and attitude yourself, they won't either...for very long. You are the leader in your practice. What you do speaks without words as to how you expect your team to work and respond to patients. Think about the mixed messages parents send to a child when the child is told not to lie, and then when the phone rings the parent says, "Tell them I'm not here." Or when the child is told that it is important and necessary to obey the law, but he witnesses the parent driving 80 in a 55 mile per hour zone. The child becomes confused and begins to wonder what really is acceptable. The next step is to try it him or herself. Remember the sayings, "What is good for the goose is good for the gander," and "Monkey see, monkey do." The same principle holds true in your office. The tone, the culture, the climate, the feeling...indeed the atmosphere, is set first by you. And your team will follow.

There is a maxim in communication that brings home the point of communication: When a person doesn't like the message or the way it is communicated, he or she sometimes crucifies the messenger. It takes time and effort to learn how to communicate well. But it's worth it. Daily headlines remind us that people today are suit-conscious...and the dental field is not exempt from those suits. Following good communication principles in your practice may well be the difference between working through a situation, or being notified that a patient has begun litigation. What's more, with great communication, you and your staff will enjoy dentistry a whole lot more. And everyone wins...you, your team and your patients!

Pay Attention to Complaints

Only five percent of patients who have a complaint will actually tell you. The other 95% are off telling an average of 11 to 16 other people. These are the statistics. The moral is that if you're not hearing any complaints you are either perfect...or you may have a problem!

Let's recognize complaints for what they can be. They are actually practice builders if you choose to look at them that way. Many individuals, however, are afraid of opening themselves to hear what the patients might have to say. The suggestion or comment box was mentioned earlier. This is an easy, painless, soft approach to getting feedback. Simply ask, *What can we do to improve our service to you?*

Patient loyalty is important; it is the core of any stable, successful practice. Very few patients have any objective way of knowing whether you did a mediocre job or a super terrific one from the clinical standpoint. Their opinion is formed based on what they feel and the interaction they have with you and your team.

When a patient calls requesting their x-rays and records be transferred to another doctor in your area (because they are leaving your practice), ask some questions to find out the reason. You'll likely learn a lot. And always add, "If we can be of service in the future, please do give us a call."

Right now take a few minutes to think about your practice and the real troublesome patients with whom you work. These are the people who tie your stomach in knots; the ones when you see their name on the daily schedule seem to put a black cloud over morning or afternoon, if not the entire day. These are the ones who drain your energy and the energy of your team. Out of your entire practice how many come to mind? One? Five? Ten? In any case, it is most likely well under 1%.

If you are still maintaining these people in your practice as patients, you are creating a stressful situation for yourself, your team, and most likely for the patient as well. It is your privilege, and perhaps we could go even further and say responsibility, to purify your practice of these patients. You do have a choice to treat or dismiss.

Summary

Most patients come to your office wanting to like and trust you, even many of those who tell you outright that they "hate dentists." When you hear this you can almost guarantee they are crying out for you to be "different" from their previous dentist or dental experiences. They don't want to be treated the way they've been treated in the past. Unfortunately, many dentists and entire teams miss this urgent plea.

> Treat the patient first, then the problem.
> When we've taken care of the person and let him or
> her know we care, then we can begin the treatment.

Patients will tell you exactly what you must do to make them happy and allow you the success you want in your work. They will tell you the truth if they know you are listening and really care. If they sense intuitively you are not, they will close down.

It is important that the entire team remembers it is up to them to establish the atmosphere. Remember ISECADA? *Interest, sincerity and enthusiasm create a desired atmosphere.* It is up to us as team members to make the first move, and sometimes the second and even the third. We get in return what we send out.

> The ultimate reward for open communication
> and honest caring is trust, and in the end
> a wonderful relationship that brings
> fulfillment and satisfaction to all involved.

If you haven't clearly defined what good service means in your practice, your chances of getting great reviews from your patients falls dramatically. A *somewhat* general definition will yield *somewhat* better results than no clarification at all, but when you have a detailed definition of what good customer service and patient relations is all about, and when it is clearly communicated, understood, accepted and believed by your team members, your chances increase tremendously of getting excellent ratings from your patients.

Your team, every single member, must be keenly aware of what good patient relations and customer service is...what it looks like in action. If they are not, it won't work. It's one thing to say courtesy and friendliness are important, but how that actually looks in behavior to one person versus another may be a totally different picture.

And remember, your team will be no more motivated to take care of the patients than they feel you are motivated to take care of them. When your employees know you really care about them, they will do what you ask...and more. They'll go the extra mile without even being asked. Everyone in your practice, beginning with the receptionist, has to sell the concept of you and your practice to the patient. There truly is no such thing as a dental team member who is not in sales!

In your quest for identifying just what good service means to your practice, ask these questions:

What would we have to do differently to make the cover of the leading dental practice trade journal or magazine?...or

What would we have to do differently to...(and name the results you want).

What makes us stand out? What could we do that we are not doing today that would make us stand out in the way of service and how we treat our patients? How are we different from other dental practices? If we don't know and can't identify why and how we are different, how can we expect our patients to?

Then determine new action based on what you hear. Today's world is such that we cannot wait to get better, to improve our practices, or even wait to move forward until other practices catch up. If you are out in front by your service distinction, but have rested on your laurels, by the time other practices catch up they will be in full gear and ready to roll right on past....and it will take you time to gear up and get the engine going again. In that span of time, however long it takes, you'll find yourself falling behind. Identify who you are and what you specifically do to build good patient relations. Pay attention to detail. Attention to detail is what will really make you stand out.

Even if you feel you don't have the room to squeeze in another patient to your practice, you must still sell people on your practice as being the very best place to come...and sell them over and over and over again. If you don't, at some point some other practice (doctor or team member) might "sell" them and win them over to their practice.

Remember, to most patients a dental practice is the same as the next...except for how they feel about it. And perceived image is their only guide.

Chapter 38

THE NEW PATIENT EXPERIENCE

The new patient experience is critical to the practice and important for each team member to understand. How the patient is greeted, treated, seated, and how this is repeated throughout the practice will determine their perception and level of expectation for future visits and whether or not they want to return. Every step along the way, every contact, whether it be over the telephone, in writing or in person, makes a difference. Each of these are, again, moments of truth.

Let's walk through the new patient experience and identify specific areas with which we should be concerned.

Phone Contact. When a patient calls your office, or if your receptionist has reached the patient as a result of outbound marketing, the entire tone of the telephone conversation is important. Answering promptly and greeting the patient in such a manner that says, *"I'm really glad you called"* is important. The receptionist should give the patient the feeling that she is listening and giving her undivided attention. The receptionist can also begin the information gathering process that will help the doctor and entire staff when the patient arrives. It may be hot buttons, fears, concerns, etc. This is information about the new patient that should be shared in the morning huddle the day of the appointment.

If there is enough time before the appointment, send the appropriate materials (patient information form, medical/dental history form) to be completed and brought to the appointment. This eliminates waiting time for the patient and allows you to be more accurate with your scheduling. New patients want information about the doctor with whom they have scheduled an appointment. Therefore a cover letter including a thank you for selecting your practice, along with a practice brochure, should accompany the patient history forms and clarify any agreements made over the phone (if you agreed to call the previous dentist to obtain chart notes and x-rays, reiterate this in the letter...if the patient was asked to bring a minimum dollar amount for the first appointment, include a reminder, etc.). The receptionist should immediately request x-rays and chart notes from the previous dentist to be included in your records.

In our practice we have developed an actual presentation packet for new patients. This packet includes: a presentation folder and five separate pages (our treatment philosophy, welcome to our practice, financial options, infection control and questions about insurance). The folder itself has two dye cuts on the bottom flap...one for Norm's card and the other for the patient's appointment card.

The presentation packet folder is also used to present the patient's treatment plan, providing them with a well-done, professional strategy, in writing, for their treatment.

First personal contact. When the patient arrives for the appointment, he should be treated as though he were a guest in your home. Addressing the patient by name and welcoming him to the practice, an introduction by the receptionist by name, and a firm handshake are all appropriate "entrance" courtesies. The patient should always, if an adult, be greeted by Mr., Mrs., or Ms., until the patient indicates they want to be addressed by their first name or nickname. It is a good idea to have a place on the information sheet for them to indicate how they would like to be addressed.

The first greeting new patients receive when walking into the practice should never be a clipboard shoved in front of them and asking them to fill it out. This will certainly diminish any positive first impression. It is cold, impersonal and makes a statement that *"You're the next number in our files. Get the paperwork done and then the doctor will see you."*

If the patient has not completed the patient information forms or has forgotten to bring them in, these must be completed. When they are completed the receptionist should double check the entire form(s) to make sure they have been completed in full. If you have a space on the form to identify how they were referred to your office, this should also be checked for completion so a thank you card can be sent to the referrer. Every line should be completed. If it becomes necessary at a later time to take collection action, incomplete information may make it difficult to track the individual for follow-up action.

It is important, even when the receptionist is on the phone or with another patient, to acknowledge the arrival of the new patient (as should be done with all patients). If she is on the phone when the patient walks through the door, all it takes is a nod and a smile that says, "I'll be with you right away." It should go without saying that if the team member is on a personal call the patient comes first and the personal call should be quickly terminated.

If you normally make coffee, tea or juice available to the patients in your practice, it is appropriate to do so at this time.

Depending upon the size of your practice, and if you have more than one person working at the front desk, a nice touch is to have one person take the patient to a separate room to set the stage and ask a few introductory questions such as:

We have a few minutes before Doctor will be in, so I'd like to go over some preliminary information with you. "

In addition to any questions the history form raises, the team member might ask:

What was it that prompted you to come see us?
Tell me a little bit about your last dentist (or dental experience).
How do you feel about your dental health?

By listening to the patient and watching non-verbal responses the team member asking the questions can learn much about your new patient in a few minutes. This can help you to quickly focus on what is important to the patient and therefore maximize treatment acceptance.

Another important point is that the patient chart should be completed as quickly as possible. Not doing so can be a time waster, patient irritant, and schedule derailer. Obviously the patient will go nowhere except sit in the reception area until the chart is ready for the assistant and doctor. Therefore, this should be a key area of concern when getting a new patient seated.

I can remember back to my days in an orthopedic practice several years ago. It became a self-played game for me to see how quickly I could get the new patient chart completed and given to the nurses to get the patient in. I was well aware that every minute it took me to complete the chart was one more minute the patient had to sit in the waiting room. I was always aware that people don't like to spend their time sitting in waiting rooms...and whether they sit a short time or a long time is all part of the first impression.

When the receptionist has completed her part in the initial greeting of the new patient, she should pass on any pertinent information she has learned about the patient to the doctor or assistant. For example, if she learns that a patient has had a terrible previous dental experience, she should relate that information. Anything that is appropriate and will give insight to the doctor and assistant should be conveyed prior to the patient being taken back to the operatory, or at least before the doctor greets the patient.

Greeting by the chairside assistant. The next logical step in the new patient flow is for the assistant to greet the new patient and take him back to the operatory. Again, this is a moment of truth. The flow from one staff member to the next should be smooth, not jerky. The patient should feel welcomed, warm, comfortable, and cared for.

The assistant should first check the chart for how the patient prefers to be addressed, whether by first name, nickname, or Mr., Mrs., etc., and then take the chart to the doctor to review prior to greeting the patient. Then the assistant should call the patient by name and welcome him or her to the practice as she introduces herself by name.

Mr. Smith? Good afternoon, Mr. Smith. My name is Sally Wright and I'm doctor's assistant. Welcome to our practice! Would you like a quick tour of our practice to see how we do things here?

A tour of the practice allows you to "sell" the practice and eliminate the patient's concerns (if any) regarding cleanliness, infection control methods, etc. and answer any questions the patient might have along the way. The assistant can actually ask a few questions as she makes the tour to relax the patient and begin building rapport.

After the tour, the patient can be seated in a treatment room until the doctor arrives. It is desirable for the assistant to remain with the patient during this time if at all possible. When you are ready to greet the patient the assistant can make the transition smoothly by saying something like:

Doctor (Name), this is Michael White. He has been referred to us by one of our favorite patients, Bob Clark. Michael, this is Dr.......

and then continue on with anything pertinent that she wants to share with you to build the bridge for communication to be picked up by you. By this time you should have already reviewed the patient chart and been informed by the receptionist of anything she knows about the patient that you should know. Any hot buttons should have been recorded on the chart such as: likes golf, auto racing, involved in specific activity or organization, avid fisherman or hunter, new dad, dental phobic...whatever it is. If a team member has learned information that is helpful to you in either communicating and bonding with the patient, or in treating the patient, you should know.

Sometimes when communication is not shared between team members the patient ends up answering the same questions over and over. This can be annoying to the patient and indicates a lack of communication in the practice.

It is important that the patient see the doctor first, rather than the hygienist. For a dentist not to diagnose periodontal disease is unprofessional, unhealthy, unethical, immoral, certainly unprofitable and most important, unfair to the patient.

Greeting by the doctor. Once you have been introduced by your assistant, welcome the new patient to your practice. Begin building rapport by mentioning something you noticed on the chart or something you were told by the receptionist. Perhaps something like,

> *Michael, I understand you were referred to us by Bob Clark. Do you work with Bob?*

> *Michael, I see you were referred to us by Bob Clark. Are you a golf enthusiast like he is?*

> *Michael, my receptionist, (name), said that you are the proud father of a new baby boy. Was this your first?*

> *Michael, I see here on your chart that you are an avid skier. Where do you do most of your skiing?*

Look for a bridge you can build on. Let the patient know you are interested in him. Ask questions. Find out about your patients. Talk with them. Learn what is important to them. Understand why they are there. After a few minutes of ice-breakers and building rapport, move into the sales process...beginning with building credibility (refer to chapter 26), identifying the need, and uncovering hot buttons. Explain the examination process and your treatment philosophy and then move into the actual examination.

The new patient exam is critical to building a solid comprehensive practice based on providing the patient with the best possible treatment options. A thorough new patient exam does many things, not the least of which is orienting a new patient to your practice philosophy and beginning to build trust. The better your new patient exam is for your patient, the more complete your treatment plan can be. When we say we are in the business of providing service, but don't follow through with a thorough exam, our integrity is in question. We are not walking our talk.

A thorough new patient examination should include the following checks:

- TMJ
- Oral cancer screen (lymph nodes, lips, buccal mucosa, floor of mouth, tongue, palate)
  Note: When you do the oral cancer exam don't be silent. Tell the patient what you are doing and why. When your findings are negative, spell it out! If you don't, they'll never know you are providing this service...and it's a positive "relief" when the findings are negative.
- Periodontal exam
- Occlusal exam (centric, protrusive, right and left lateral, check for balancing and working interferences)
- Chart restorations and current condition of teeth
- Take x-rays, if necessary (assistant to take)...determined by what has been taken by previous doctor and when, and presenting symptoms at this time
- Other: diagnostic models, intraoral photographs, etc.

If you have an intraoral video camera, the new patient exam is a great place to introduce it to the patient. This may be the first time the patient has ever had the opportunity to see what the mouth actually looks like from every angle and it will help anchor the problems you identify.

Following the physical exam, determine what is needed next. Perhaps the patient needs to begin seeing the hygienist for periodontal therapy, root planing, a simple prophy....or perhaps immediate treatment is needed to deal with a critical situation. Whatever it is, explain the next steps to the patient. Let the patient know you need some time to study the radiographs (study models, etc.) and determine the best treatment plan for his/her situation. It is best to schedule the return visit to present the treatment plan as soon after the initial visit as possible. Anything longer than a week is questionable.

Finally, as you end the first appointment, accompany the patient to the front desk and let the receptionist know when you want the patient scheduled.

(Receptionist's name), I'd like to see Michael again for a treatment plan consultation within 3-7 days.

Turning to the patient:

Michael, it was a pleasure to meet you and I'll look forward to seeing you in the next few days. Thank you, once again, for selecting our office. We look forward to serving you.

Front Desk Completes the First Appointment. Again, we never get a second chance to make a good first impression. Every step along the way, care should be taken to give the patient undivided attention, to listen, and to respond to the patient's needs, questions and concerns. Now, as the patient is ready to schedule the next appointment and leave the office, the final impression is just as important as every other moment of truth. In fact, it can be the most important because it is the last impression the patient has as he leaves the office.

The receptionist needs to: (1) schedule the consultation appointment, (2) again welcome the patient to the practice and thank him for coming in and (3) remain warm, friendly, smile, and let the patient feel he is truly welcomed. After the patient leaves a thank you note should be sent to the *referring* person. A welcome card or letter should also go to the *new patient* following the appointment.

A follow up telephone call to the patient by the receptionist is another way of anchoring the new relationship, especially if there has been emergency treatment provided the patient.

Michael, I'm calling to see how you are doing? (If the patient gives a great response the receptionist can continue:)

I'm really please to hear that...that's exactly how we want you to feel. Michael, I'd like to offer you the opportunity to refer any friends or relatives, people like yourself, to our practice if they are looking for a great doctor and a caring staff. We will welcome any referral you make.

Or, if the patient was concerned about pain and was a bit phobic, but says the experience in your office was great:

That's great to hear, Michael. I know you had some concerns. Perhaps you have friends or family members who don't know how dentistry has changed. We'd welcome your referral of these people and we'll give them the same care all our patients have come to expect and enjoy from us!

We often miss the prime opportunity of gaining referrals from new patients. Normally only 20% of the patients in a practice will refer, and new patients will generally refer more than long-established patients *if they liked the experience in your office.* Therefore, be sure to ask for referrals early in your relationship with a new patient, as well as throughout the time he or she is in your practice.

Treatment Plan Consultation. When the patient returns, it is important to recap and build the patient's emotional level to where it was when he left the first appointment. Review what was originally identified, what the patients concerns, needs and wants were. At this time, in addition to presenting the treatment plan orally, give it to the patient in written form. A written treatment plan eliminates confusion and misunderstanding. They also reduce the possibility of a patient later saying, "I had no idea the treatment was going to be this expensive" or "I remember you telling me it was going to be___$, not ___$."

Before we began putting treatment plans in writing in our practice we had this confusion. Norm would present a treatment plan, perhaps with a range of, say, $3,200 to $4,000, depending upon certain factors or what was actually discovered when the treatment was begun. What do you suppose the patient tended to remember? That's right, the $3,200. Now, with treatment plans in writing there can be no confusion. It also states that this is an estimate and the actual fee may vary depending upon what the actual condition is once treatment is begun.

Shocking as it may seem, as many as 50% of all dental offices do not do treatment plans! It is the responsibility of the dentist to educate the patient as to his or her oral health condition...and what is necessary in order to restore and maintain good dental health. The sales process, including the new patient experience, is designed to do just that.

Give people the very best. Give them alternatives, too, if appropriate, but do present to them what you would want in your mouth or your family's. Don't prejudge what you believe your patients can afford. Also realize from a business standpoint that it is not necessary to play banker and finance the larger treatment plans "in house." It is, however, important to provide the patient with various options for payment, such as check, cash, Visa, Master Card, Discover Card, American Express, or various healthcare credit cards. The more options you have, the easier it will be for the patient to move forward with treatment.

Post Treatment Consultation. Following the actual treatment plan completion, it is a good idea to consult with your patient in your private office once again. Review what you originally indicated needed to be done and the condition of the patient's mouth, what you actually accomplished with the treatment, what your responsibility is, what the patient's responsibility is, what interval is required because of the patient's oral health condition for continuing care visits, and what problems need to be monitored.

This completes the new patient cycle for this patient. Every phase indicated above is a part of the new patient cycle, and the new patient experience. The experience involves much more than the dental treatment itself, as we can see Building the relationship with the patient, by every member of the team, is important; a comprehensive exam is necessary for restorative success; and communicating with the patient is critical to building trust and educating for future care.

In the end, the entire process of dealing with the patient, from the first telephone call to the very last time the patient has any contact with your office, is important in establishing, building, and maintaining a good, solid, healthy relationship with you and your dental team. And understanding all that goes into patient relations and customer service is critically important to that process.

People don't care how much you know until they know how much you care. When you have a caring team, one that truly cares for each and every patient, and is concerned about each and every action or behavior and the impact it will have on the patient, then you will have a practice that is well known for good patient relations. When your patients like, really like, the experience of being in your office, of doing business with you, then you will have done a great job of marketing. You'll also have the distinction that sets you apart from every other practice in town. And you'll certainly have the peace of mind that comes from service to your fellow human beings.

Chapter 39

THE JOURNEY CONTINUES

As we move into the new millenium, the 21st century, it is obvious that much has changed in our industry, in our society, and indeed in our world. But some things haven't changed...the need and the desire to build dental practices that are productive and satisfying, and that allow balance, harmony, and a sense of fulfillment in our lives.

Emerson said, "Shallow men believe in luck, wise and strong men in cause and effect." There is an investment to be made for success, as there has always been. The critical question to ask yourself is, "Am I willing to make that investment? Am I willing to do what I need to do today to move in the direction of my dreams, my desires...to journey forward toward the practice I really want to have? Or will I settle for the *easy methods* and sacrifice those dreams and desires...settling for just good enough or mediocrity?

Dentistry, regardless of the obstacles and challenges that lie ahead, has never been better. I believe that dentists today can become even more productive than in the past and capitalize on the demand for dental care. Although the need for some services has seemed to decrease, the need for other dental services is on the rise. The question, then, is not whether there are good times ahead for dentistry, but whether you and your practice will adapt to the changing expectations and methods of practicing. The practices that don't will fall behind, and the practices that do will experience the best that is yet to come..

Leaders are never content with the status quo. They know there is always a new path to forge, a refinement to be made. They know that for every cause, there is an effect...and every effect has its cause.

Take a moment before you put this book down and ask yourself what one step you can take that would contribute the most to your journey at this time...then commit to taking it. Be directed...know what you want and go forward with that focus, that vision. Love every part of your life and your practice.

So, my friend, this book must end not with my words, but with your commitment to the principles and to the process. I call you my friend because I have poured out my heart in the pages of this book, in the hope that I might touch yours.

We've come a long way together, but now you must continue the journey...your journey...to the life and the practice you have always wanted to have. May God bless you and be with you every step of the way.

APPENDIX A

Interview Questions

It is helpful to remember that in every interview there are "two" applicants...the real applicant and the applicant she chooses to present (or as she feels the interviewer would like her to be). It is the responsibility of the interviewer to distinguish between the two, and good questions and questioning technique will help accomplish this objective.

When conducting the interview, be aware of regulations established by The Privacy Act, The Civil Rights Act and the guidelines of the Human Rights Commission. By law you may not discriminate against those with disabilities in regard to any employment practices, including hiring practices, if such individuals meet the skill, education, experience, and other job-related requirements of the position, and if such persons can, with or without reasonable accommodation, perform the essential duties of the position.

Be aware that questions during the interview process may not be asked if they refer to disabilities, marital status, race, national origin, age and sex. Questions regarding religious affiliations, religious denomination or religious holidays observed are also not allowed. Other questions best not asked which could create legal issues are:

Were you born in the United States?
Do you have children (or what are their names or ages)?
Are you single, married, divorced or separated?
Have you ever been treated for the following illnesses?
Do you wish to be addressed as Ms., Miss or Mrs.?
What clubs, societies and organizations do you belong to?

You can ask applicants if they smoke. There are several questions that can be asked that give you great information that you couldn't ask for directly, but are still legal. An example of these are:

- Mary Jane, we have a very busy, fast paced practice. This means that the person we hire must be able to keep up with a fast pace and be on their feet all day. How comfortable do you feel standing on your feet for a full day?

  Here you are trying to get to whether or not the applicant has back or other health problems that would make it difficult for her to keep pace. Notice that the question doesn't say, "Can you stand....?" This calls for a yes or no and the applicant can easily figure that you want a yes. By asking the "how" questions, it calls for some explanation. It will be less likely the applicant can answer without giving you some clue to the "real" answer.

- Mary Jane, have you ever used another name?

  Here you are getting information for checking references...and it will give you a clue as to their current marital status.

- Here's a question to find out whether or not an individual can be at work regularly during your time frames, and yet not require you to ask a question regarding younger children (which is a violation of the regulations).

  Mary Jane, we require all our employees to be here and ready to begin work promptly at 7:00 with no exceptions. We begin our day with the morning huddle to get us all moving in the same direction and set the tone for the day. Also, we normally schedule until 4:00, but it is rare that we finish with patients and clean-up until 4:30 or 4:45. How will meeting these times consistently work for you?

Work Experience/History

It is obvious this is an integral part of the interview process. Knowing the applicant's past work record, experience level and work history is important.

- One area we want to discuss today is your work experience. Would you tell me about your present (or last) position.

- What were your major responsibilities on your last job?

- In your last position, what were some of the things you spent the most time on? How much time did you spend on each?

- How many days of work would you say you missed last year?

How applicant feels about her work/job
Knowing how the applicant feels about her work is important, in addition to knowing what the work history has been.

- Why did you leave (or...are you leaving) your last position? *Always look for more than one reason for a voluntary resignation.*

- What regrets do you have (did you have) in leaving your last position?

- What did you like most about your position with...? Least?

- What was the most difficult part of your work? Why?

- If you could have made any changes, what would they have been?

- How would you describe your ideal work day?

- What are some of the things relating to your work that you feel you have done particularly well?

- Where do you feel you have achieved the greatest success (or progress) in your last position? Why?

- What new work-related skills or capabilities have you developed over the past year?

- What are some of the problems you encounter in doing your

job? What frustrates you the most? How do you handle them?

- In what ways do you feel your present job has developed you to take on even greater responsibilities?

- What is your greatest frustration (or disappointment) in your current position? What are some of your reasons for feeling this way?

- Do you consider your progress in your last position representative of your ability? Why or why not?

- How do you feel about irregular work hours? Overtime?

- How would you describe the way you respond under pressure/stress?

- What would you identify as the three most important functions that a (hygienist, assistant, receptionist, treatment coordinator, etc.) performs?

Career Objectives
It is important to know the applicant's career objectives. What is she looking for and what does she wish to avoid in her career/ position?

- What do you expect to accomplish in the next two years?

- Where do you see yourself five years from now?
  How will you make that a reality?

- What do you feel you need to know in order to determine whether or not you could be successful in the position we have open?

- What are your most important considerations in making your career choice?

- What things would you like to avoid in your position? Why?

- What would you like from your next position that you didn't get from your last one?

- How would you describe your over-all career objectives? What, outside your job, have you done or plan to do that will help you achieve this objective?

- What are your salary (income) expectations? What would you consider satisfactory salary (income) progress over the next couple years?

How applicant feels about people

An important part in determing career success potential is knowing the way the applicant feels about people...both co-workers and supervisors. The following questions will help explore this important area.

- How do you feel about working with close supervision? Little supervision?

- How do you feel about structure in your work setting?

- How often are you approached by other people for advice? How do you handle it?

- How would you describe your last supervisor/doctor? When you had disagreements, what would they generally be about? How do you feel about the way you were treated by your supervisor/doctor? How did your supervisor/doctor help you to develop your potential? What did your supervisor/doctor feel you did particularly well? What were his/her major criticisms? How do you feel about those criticisms?

- How would you describe the kind of people you like to work with best?
How would you describe the kind of people with whom you least like to work?

- Who, in your last position, would you say you got along least with? What did you do about it?

- Relating to serving the patient, what does quality service mean to you? What, specifically, would let me know that quality service is being provided a patient?

- Can you give me some examples of times when you, personally, went the extra mile for the patients in providing quality patient service?

- Sometimes we can be thrown off by difficult patients. What would you do if you had an unhappy, or even irate, patient?

How applicant feels about herself
How the applicant feels about herself plays a big role in determining how stable or secure she will feel, how she will relate to others, how she will be able to accept criticism and suggestions. To learn more about this area, the following questions will help.

- How would you describe yourself?

- Would you tell me something about yourself?
Note: If you ask this question or one related and the applicant tells you something about him/herself that brings up the discriminatory subject (such as married, about spouse, children, etc.) you can ask specific questions about that issue, as long as the applicant was the one who brought it up. You cannot be the first to bring it up.

- If our employees were to ask me what they should know about you in order to work well with you, what would I tell them?

- If, after completing all the interviews, I had three people who had the same experience level, good references and compa-

rable education, and you were one of the three...why
do you feel my best decision would be to hire you?

- How are you different now from when you began your last
  position?

- What two things drain your energy the most?
  What two things energize you the most?

- In the last year, what was your greatest non-work accomplishment?

- In the last year, what gave you the greatest encouragement?

- What was the most discouraging thing that happened in the
  last year? How did you respond to it?

- How do you motivate yourself when you are "down?"

- What do you feel are your greatest strengths?
  How would they contribute to our practice?

- What do you consider to be your greatest areas for
  improvement?

Related to your practice
It is helpful to know what the applicant knows about your practice and whether there is a real desire to work specifically with your practice vs. simply looking anywhere for a "job." Here are some helpful questions to elicit this information.

- What sparked your interest in our practice? Or what about
  our ad attracted you?

- What can our practice do for you?

- Concerning our practice, what do you bring to us that is
  different than any other (hygienist, assistant, bookkeeper,
  treatment coordinator, etc) we might hire?

<u>Other</u>

- If you were hiring someone for this position, what (qualities) would you look for?

- If I criticized you and you felt it was unjust, or I snapped at you, how would you respond?

- How would you describe your ideal philosophy of the dental practice with which you want to be involved?

- What are the most important qualities you are looking for in the dental practice of your choice?

APPENDIX B

Conducting a Telephone Reference Check

It should be remembered that a reference check is a mini-interview. One way to begin the telephone interview is by simply identifying yourself and stating the purpose of your call. For example:

Good morning, (name). My name is (your name) and I'm a dentist in(city).(Name of applicant) has applied for employment with us as a (name of position). May I ask you a few questions concerning her employment with you?"

As in any interview, it is best to begin with the less sensitive topics and as rapport is established to move on to the more difficult, sensitive areas. With this in mind, an appropriate place to begin is to check employment dates.

Employment dates are important because they help you account for time. Any time unaccounted for on the applicant's record may hide an experience that could disqualify the applicant from further employment consideration. It would be unwise to hire someone when you know there are significant periods of time during which her activities or whereabouts are unknown. Additionally, many times an applicant who wants to hide an unpleasant experience will try to do so by juggling employment, school, and military service dates. Therefore, checking the actual dates may prove to be very beneficial.

There are two ways to inquire about employment dates...one correct and one incorrect. Here are examples of both.

Incorrect: *(Name) says she was employed by you from January 15, 1994 to April 23, 1994. Is this correct?*

This approach is incorrect because it begs the question and gives the interviewee a ready-made answer, especially handy if he/she doesn't want to bother looking up the correct dates. If he relies on memory alone, his "yes" answer may simply mean the person was employed, but not necessarily that the dates are accurate.

Correct: From your records, can you tell me when (name) began employment with your practice, and when she left?

Here the interviewee must give his/her own answer. If he consults his records the answer should be accurate.

It is natural to move into a discussion of job responsibilties and general work performance at this point. The following questions are examples that will lead you into a discussion of these areas:

What was her position in your practice?
What were her duties in that position?
How would you rate her performance in work volume?
How would you rate her performance in work quality?
How much supervision did she require?
How would you describe her attitude?
Did her conduct ever require any disciplinary measures?
How would you rate her performance compared with the performance of others who had similar responsibilities...or with others who have held that position either before or since?
What was her income level when she left?
How punctual was this person?
What was her attendance record?
What do you feel are her greatest strengths?
What do you feel are her greatest weaknesses?

Ask additional questions relating specifically to the job itself, such as, for the hygienist:
How would you describe her approach to patient education?
Her willingness to work with the team?
Did she require an assistant?
What was her daily production?

It is also important to fully understand why the applicant left previous jobs. In most cases, there is usually more than one reason behind her leaving, and the lead-in question should stress this idea:

> Would you tell me the circumstances leading to (name) termination?

> Would you consider her for rehire?

If the applicant was fired:

> Would you tell me the reasons for her termination?

There are a couple questions that may disclose a practice that was never mentioned by the applicant during the interview. In many cases, a "voluntary oversight" such as this may be prompted by the applicant's desire to hide an unsatisfactory experience.

> Could you tell me the name of the doctor (name) worked for prior to working with you?
> And the name of the doctor she worked for after leaving your practice?

Finally, one final interview question will give the reference source an opportunity to provide any additional information he feels may be pertinent. This often brings out in the open significant information that might otherwise have been overlooked.

> Is there anything else you can tell me about (name)?

The Principled Practice

A Comprehensive Guide to the Non-Clinical Aspects of Dentistry

ORDERING INFORMATION

Additional books can be ordered for $49.95 each. Include $4.95 for shipping and handling for the first book, and $2.50 for each additional book in the same order. Send check or money order to:

Soaring Horizons® Productions
P. O. Box 25406
Portland, Oregon 97225
or call
1-800-5-CHERYL

Allow 2-3 weeks for delivery.

FOR FURTHER INFORMATION ABOUT CHERYL...

If you would like to find out more about Cheryl's speaking, training and practice development consulting services, please write or call her at:

The Cheryl Matschek Company
P. O. Box 25406
Portland, Oregon 97225
1-800-5-CHERYL or FAX 503-292-2752